Sticking It To Cancer

Sticking It To Cancer

Joana Montenegro

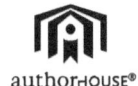

authorHOUSE®

AuthorHouse™
1663 Liberty Drive
Bloomington, IN 47403
www.authorhouse.com
Phone: 1-800-839-8640

First published by AuthorHouse   11/03/2011

ISBN: 978-1-4678-6965-2 (sc)
ISBN: 978-1-4678-6964-5 (ebk)

Printed in the United States of America

I love you when you're happy
I love you when you're sad
I love you when you're naughty
I love you when you're mad

July 21st 2010 is a date I'll never forget. I was minding my own business, obsessing over all the silly things we obsess over, beating myself up over all the silly things we beat ourselves up over and somehow had spent the past 37 years of my life convinced I was going to live forever. And that's when I got the phone call. I was in my office wearing my favorite heels and on my way to some mega important meeting when the phone rang. I was about to walk out but recognized the number as being my clinic so I picked up without even bothering to sit down. And that's when my life changed in a single minute: "Is this Joana? Well, it turns out you have cancer in the left breast, at the 11 o'clock position and it has spread to your lymph nodes. What number can our surgeon call you at?". After giving her my cell phone number I walked out of my office and towards my car. All I could think was that I was going to die and leave behind a 6 year old daughter (Lucy) who I adored, a 3 year old son (Daniel) who was the apple of my eye and they would never remember me. As I got on the elevator a huge wave of relief came over me though. I looked back a numerous difficult decisions I had made in my life and realized I had no regrets. Thank God for that. No regrets. I didn't regret any of my tough choices and hadn't really understood that until I was staring at my mortality as the elevator took me down to the exit of the building.

I went to the Mayo Clinic in Rochester, MN to be in some clinical trials. This first and most important was a series of 12 weekly chemo treatments followed by a bilateral mastectomy with reconstruction and finished up with a second round of 4 chemotherapy treatments and 25 radiation sessions. A very long marathon!

So, my husband Steve and I gathered the kids and embarked as a family on this journey. We were recently married and blending our respective children into a cohesive family of 6 when our lives were turned upside down.

But we're all better for it and I am thankful for the opportunity to grow up, discover what's really important and stick it to cancer!

This is the journal I kept hoping that one day our children might be able to read it and understand what actually happened . . .

Friday the 13th . . . . !

Aug 13, 2010 1:53am

Friday the 13th is a VERY important day because it's Lucy's 6th birthday! She's growing up so fast.

I also get my second chemo dose which I am oddly looking forward to. Just knowing those drugs are killing the cancer, making it smaller and preventing it from spreading makes me feel good. And after my first round I know that I can handle the side effects . . .

In the next couple of weeks, my hair will fall out—I will need to get used to that! But I have some really cute head scarves and hats so I'll be set!

Second chemo round . . .

Aug 14, 2010 12:11am

I just got my second dose of chemotherapy today—good to know all that poison is running around in here getting those cancer cells (and my hair!).

The experience wasn't bad the first time, everyone is so nice but this time I was even more relaxed. I think I managed to take 3 shallow breaths as they put the IV in. PROGRESS! (I hate needles, I hate needles, I hate needles).

But they don't just give me a cocktail of chemo drugs, they also give me steroids. Thank God for steroids! Seriously. I feel great, could eat a horse, no side effects at least not yet, but in 2 days I'll feel like a train ran me over.

Tomorrow I'm going to hang out with the hubby and kids, go to a cancer yoga class because my brain is going to help the drugs as best it can and generally eat everything in site.

Take care everyone! Thanks for the encouraging notes. In a year, I will thank you all for contributing to my recovery.

Bye-bye Hair . . .

Aug 14, 2010 10:13pm

I hear one of the hardest parts for women being treated with breast cancer is the hair loss. I've never been 'into' my hair, never spent time styling it or coloring it, but now that I know I'll lose it in the next week: I'm suddenly attached to it!

What I don't want to have happen is one of my kids to walk into my bedroom one morning to cuddle with me for a bit and find clumps of hair on my pillow. So tomorrow, after Lucy's birthday party, I'm having the kids help me shave it off. We'll have a "Bye Bye Hair" party. I'm determined to NOT let cancer do things to me if I can control the event myself. So that's what we'll do tomorrow.

That aside, I'm feeling very well. I spend a ton of time outside, fresh air does wonders!

Next week I have a bunch of appointments but Monday is light so I'm taking Lucy for a girls day out down at the Mayo. She really wants to go see this place I keep going to. She and I will drive down together, I'll show her the piano where someone is always playing tunes, the cool big windows all around the waiting areas and the friendly people. We'll go to a wig/scarf store together and get tips on make-up during chemo (she'll LOVE that!!). We'll go for lunch at one of the cute diners with patio seating and then return home. She'll love it, I'm sure. Quality time with my princess.

Take care all!

Hair came off!

Aug 15, 2010 9:07pm

I'm posting a picture taken right after Steve shaved my head—in the next few days it should just naturally and quickly fall out.

This was definitely not easy and I do confess to crying in the shower as I rinsed to get all the hair off after the cut. Lucy and Daniel were not swayed a whole lot other than Lucy once again asking me WHY my medicine is going to make my hair fall out. That is probably the part that disturbs her the most so I'm pleased that I made the decision to slowly make it shorter and shorter for them to adjust.

Ok—next hurdle is seeing the tiny hairs fall out and then get used to people staring at me.

Getting a port in tomorrow

Aug 16, 2010 9:52pm

Tomorrow I go in for an outpatient surgery where a power port will be put into my chest. Essentially it's a line that goes directly into a vein in my neck through which all chemo can be delivered, any blood draws taken and any medication provided through this thing sitting right under my skin. So no more IV's and no more needles other than the one used to access the port sitting under my skin.

It's going to make life a lot easier on me needle wise but the whole procedure is disturbing to think about. Threading a tube into a big vein in my neck . . . yuck.

They do it all under conscious sedation which I've had before. You don't remember a thing after and it feels like someone injected 5 margaritas into you all at once. Apparently last time I got this type of sedation I spent the entire time trying to order McDonalds from the nurses. I'm sure I'll embarrass myself in some similar fashion tomorrow. I'll let ya know!

Take care

The Power Port is now online!

Aug 17, 2010 8:40pm

Ok—so the stupid power port in now under my skin and jammed into a vein in my neck. I'm slowly turning into the bionic woman . . . . fake vein in the form of a power port and pretty soon fake boobs. I should give into Lucy's wishes and get the wig . . .

"How did the actual procedure go?" I hear you ask . . .

Well, I couldn't eat or drink until 10:30 am and did I mention they give me steroids with the chemo? Steroids make me HUNGRY! (I've actually gained 7 lbs these past few weeks). I was HUNGRY!

The prep takes a long time. First the nurse wants to make sure you are fully aware of the fact that a 2mm diameter tube will get shoved into your neck vein. They explain it over and over in disgustingly graphic detail . . . I GET IT ALREADY! Sheesh!

Then comes what was supposed to be my last IV. It took 4 tries. FOUR TRIES! It kept popping out of my arm.

The funniest part—well at least from my perspective—was when I suddenly said "Yea, I think I changed my mind and don't want a port anymore". Hahahhaha . . . . technically they have to let me go back home if I refuse the procedure. The woman's expression was priceless! She laughed afterwards thankfully. Note to self: always be nice to the lady with the needle and the drugs.

Anyway, I get wheeled into the operating room and suddenly felt those 5 margaritas going right into my blood stream. The last thing I remember was saying "Give my another margarita because I can still think coherently".

The funniest part—this time according to the nurses—was that I spent the entire time telling them I was going to get meatloaf and mashed potatoes! I swear! I did it again! Food on the brain . . . .

Getting Ready for long day tomorrow

Aug 19, 2010 11:22am

Today is the first day I have had the time to just stay home since the diagnosis! I'm still going to sneak Lucy out of school to watch a girly movie on the couch but nevertheless I'm going to make an effort to rest today. Tonight we are going down to Rochester because Friday will be brutal! I start with a PET scan at 6:30 am, blood draws, another biopsy for the clinical trial folks to get more data and finally chemo until 5:30 pm. Whew!

I'm wearing hats and scarves all the time now even though my hair is still hanging on. When I put the head scarf on Daniel always says "Mommy, you go be pirate now? You go be pirate?". He's so cute!

Getting Chemo—week 3

Aug 20, 2010 5:16pm

Whew! What a day!

We spent the night here because my first appointment was at 6:30 am but neither one of us slept well because the hotel I picked kinda sucked. I swear our room was the size of a cubicle. Literally. If Steve rolled over in bed he'd risk rolling out of the window—no joke.

We trek over to the clinic at the crack of dawn to my PET scan which takes about 2 hours. They inject me with some radioactive thing then I need to sit in the dark for an hour so it can get into my cells. The guy giving me the shot (yes, another shot!) was chatting with me and I mentioned he was really good at giving painless shots, and that he should go work in the chemo ward. He shivered and said he doesn't mess with chemo drugs . . . "that stuff is poison, I go nowhere near it!!". Nice . . . .

After my hour sitting in silence and not allowed to move much, I then lie on my back with my arms above my head and am passed in and out of this huge tube for 40 minutes . . . also without being allowed to move. They threaten you with "IF you move even in the slightest, we need to do it all over again!!!!". Naturally, around minute 3 of the scan your nose itches. And it only gets worse when your arms go totally numb. Well, that's not entirely true, there's also a sharp shooting pain down your arms into the small of your back. But remember: don't move!

After the PET scan came another blood draw to make sure I have enough white blood cells to go ahead with the chemo. Remember the port I put in? The port from which they can draw blood, do chemo, etc without sticking my veins? Well . . . . I didn't let them use the port and made them stick me instead. I know, I know. I'm nuts. I go through all that pain and surgery only to freak out on the poor nurses and NOT let them use the port. I told the nurse I'm totally irrational and since I've come to terms with that, she should too. After that, it was time for a third biopsy. As part of the clinical trial, I need to let them take samples to track the impact of the new drugs. I had to keep thinking I'm doing this for all the little girls out there so they don't need to go through quite the ordeal we do today. Luckily I had the BEST radiologist this time. He was awesome! I barely felt the needle (yes, another few shots) and he was great during the procedure. But here's the thing . . . . I really had to try hard not to laugh. He's a dead ringer for Peter Sellers. DEAD RINGER! I kept having all these flashes of the old Pink Panther movies and all the other hilarious movies he was in. I know for a fact I smiled WAY too wide at him and stifled at least 2 giggles.

And now here I am, getting my chemo. I caved and let the nurse use my port this time. I nearly broke Steve's hand as she gave me the tiny poke and I have to confess it's better (and safer) than the IV's. But man, was I stressed as she was putting it in.

By the way—the results of my tests came back already because of course the Mayo is AWESOME. My white blood cells are still really good and the PET scan shows a 2/3 decrease in cancer cell activity. TAKE THAT CANCER!

Waiting for Godot

Aug 21, 2010 6:23pm

Last night we could tell a lot of my hair was coming out if we kinda pulled at it. So I expected it to be gone today but nope . . . a lot seems to be falling out but it's not really made a dent in how I look yet. Argh! All this waiting for the darn hair to make up it's mind and just be gone. It's almost more irritating to have this short stubble catching in my hats.

I'm a bit tired today from the chemo. That stuff really knocks you out! But after a nap, I'm ready for a walk and some QT with the hubby!

Better Day!

Aug 22, 2010 10:53am

I slept for 10 hours and feel a lot better today. I think having woken up yesterday at 4 am was part of my feeling extra tired.

Steve made an awesome breakfast and we're ready to hit our long errand list!

These chemo side effects are just bizarre let me tell ya. Everything tastes the same (a mixture of numb and metallic), I have odd body aches and feel pretty weak. It definitely does it's job though! Go chemo, go!

Have a peaceful happy day! I know I will!

Kinda boring day . . .

Aug 23, 2010 7:12pm

Today I got to drop the car off at the repair shop—water pump leaking. Steve had the other car so I walked back home; about a 45 minute walk back. It felt really good (and hot!) but totally knocked me out for the afternoon. I guess it's true about conserving energy! I did enjoy the walk though.

Tomorrow I need to be smarter about what I do instead of a 2 hour nap on the couch like today. I don't have a car so driving to the lake or meeting people to chat is out of the question for a few days . . . . crumbs . . .

I'm a little disappointed I was so tired today. I'm pretty determined to not let the chemo impact my daily life a whole lot. Tomorrow will be different!!!

Oh—and my hair keeps falling out by the pound but it doesn't look any different yet. Not sure why I'm fixated on the hair thing but I want it to make up it's mind and move on. Chemo goes until end of October so I have many weeks of this before surgery.

In my mind I'm aiming for July 21st 2011; the year mark of my diagnosis. I'm curious what the world will be like for me then. All done with this is my goal!

Peace all

Going to be a good day!

Aug 24, 2010 11:18am

The interesting thing cancer does to you is strip away all the exterior indications of who you are (or were). Obviously there is a drastic physical appearance change with hair loss, a few subtle skin changes and some generic pain that takes away your energy. So learning to live with limited reserves is going to be key. Not looking like I used to takes some getting used to also . . . I have had to drop the labels I had for myself regarding my physical appearance. Surgery will elevate that to a new level, I have no doubt.

And then there's the other label we carry around which is "what we do for a living". I don't know how quickly I can go back to work and to being the Operations Business Manager I used to be . . . come to think of it, I might not even go back to that title when I go back to General Mills.

So the question I've been left with is: "I am a . . . .".

I'm certainly not interested in being "a breast cancer patient". It's just something going on right now, but it's certainly never going to be elevated to a position of defining me.

Questions, questions . . . .

As much as it ticks me off to have to address these issues right now because I'm a firm believer that ignorance is bliss (kidding!). I'm sure it's going to be another gift cancer gives me and that is to figure out who I am independently of the trappings of mundane life. Lucky me . . . .

It's Daniel's Turn to be Sick

Aug 25, 2010 11:08am

Well, today it's all about Daniel Afonso. I woke up at 3 am and discovered Daniel in our bed fast asleep next to me. Nothing unusual there but I'd say I started to suspect something was up when he vomited all over himself and the bedspread . . . mmm . . . . my keen maternal instinct told me he might be sick . . .

Here's the pattern my wonderful 2 year old is stuck in:

1. Nap for 20 minutes

2. Wake up with a confused look on his face

3. Throw up all over himself and me, mostly missing the huge towel I set aside for this precise occasion

4. Tell me "I got owie in my tummy"

5. Throw up some more while pushing the towel out of his face (at this point I'm trying to contain the spill and doing as good a job as BP did in the Gulf)

6. Look up at me with those big huge eyes and pouts (this means he's feeling better)

7. Get changed into a new t-shirt (I change too . . . he always nails me!)

8. Display a huge smile and say "Mommy, I want eat now!"

9. Mommy feeds him knowing it's a big mistake

10. Daniel plays for a bit

11. Return to step 1.

I realize that while on chemo I really can't get sick myself but this is my little boy we're talking about here! I have to cuddle with him when he's sick! It's a physical impossibility for a mom to not take care of her sick child, I just hope it's not catching.

On the chemo side effect front: my energy is coming back thankfully. I need to have a good 4th chemo cycle—kids home all week!

Why Did I get Cancer?

Aug 26, 2010 10:24pm

One of the questions that has popped up for several people is whether I have been able to give my cancer diagnosis some meaning. The classic "Why me?" Interestingly enough I didn't have to give that one a whole lot of thought and pondering. I was clear on that answer from minute one.

Whether you believe in karma, God, destiny, one thing I know for sure: people are not punished so this didn't happen as a means of punishment. Bad things do happen to people, but I also believe there is some force that assigns these situations in a thoughtful way and for a reason. I think it makes sense that I would be given something that I can handle. Perhaps someone else was spared by my getting the cancer. Someone without a wonderful husband, without wonderful kids and without all of you out there. I've started to see this breast cancer as something we are all fighting together. You and me. Those of you that post regularly, those of you that don't love the blogging so you send me separate emails or phone calls and those of you that fear "bothering me" but still follow and send good vibes! We are all together beating this thing, right? :o) Thank you!

So maybe we spared someone less fortunate from dealing with what is not the hardest thing I've had to manage in my life but definitely comes in second.

And then there is all that having cancer has done for my personal growth; something I'd not likely be able to come to by myself. I don't think I ever truly realized how we are all connected and all rely on each other . . . and how that's a good thing! I've been so touched by the support.

I have also come to terms with the fact that we truly don't have control over our lives. Those of us with an illness are as uncertain of tomorrow as those of us without some diagnosis. We are mostly convinced of things like "I'll be there for my grandkids" or "When I'm 65 I'm moving to Florida" or even "Next year I'll do better at . . .". But the reality is no one knows that will happen for sure. The truth is, the only thing that exists for any of us is this present moment and nothing else. All plans in the future are merely plans but they really mean very little. So if we live in the future, live thinking "When this happens, then I'll do that", we are living in a bit of an illusion.

Now don't get me wrong, I fully plan on being there for my grandkids! And I plan on turning 65! But this realization has changed how I approach the present moment and how much value I place in it. Being a good mother for my kids doesn't mean I'll be there for their graduations because right now they are not graduating. Being a good mother means exclusively giving them what they need today and what comes after, comes after. But for now, I am thankful for the life I have today. And I believe I was probably not a terrible choice for the next woman getting breast cancer since I have all of you right here with me. All of this is why me.

A Third of the Way Done!

Aug 27, 2010 1:28pm

Round #4 of chemo will be done in 30 minutes. Only 8 to go this round! . . . not that I'm counting or anything . . .

The good news today was seeing the oncologist nurse to get the tumor measured and I now proceed to quote: "That's some impressive shrinkage!". It's way smaller! TAKE THAT! HA!

Busy Weekend

Aug 29, 2010 6:04pm

It's been one crazy weekend! Lots of kids activities, lots of fun and no time to rest. We spent the day at the Water Park chasing 9 kids around for Anthony's birthday party and now we're all back home and exhausted.

It's a little odd to watch people see me with Lucy and Daniel, notice my head scarf and guess at the lack of hair and then either avert their eyes or look at me with sorrow. It's hard to see those reminders of the cancer and it's severity. I guess at the same time I was feeling those sharp twinges while I was there—twinges which mean the tumor is getting smaller! The nurse told me those "pains" are the tumor getting pulled as it gets smaller.

One day at a time . . .

Energy Back!

Aug 31, 2010 9:27am

Ok—I'm feeing close to normal again. My energy level is back up to manageable!

I do have a few random thoughts today:

1. For all those men out there who are bald . . . . now i understand your plight! It's * * * cold without hair!!!!

2. After participating in another new imaging trial yesterday, and seeing just how good breast imaging COULD be: mammograms SUCK!

3. I miss wine. The chemo sort of wrecks my taste buds and the biggest victim has been booze . . .

4. I don't understand how two small children can generate so much noise.

Have a great day! Take a second to give someone a hug.

Love the new car!

Sep 1, 2010 8:18pm

It's so great when the chemo symptoms are mostly gone! I have energy, am in a great mood and sometimes sort of forget I have cancer. To be honest I'm still taken aback when I look in the mirror and I don't have the long hair I used to see! But people tell me I look good, my eyes still sparkle and I seem "normal".

Oh and the hair thing . . . I shaved it off with a blade . . . . and it's sort of coming back! I know a lot of it seemed to be falling out which drove me to just shave it clean. Well . . . now it's returning. Good grief! Make up your mind already?!!???!!

Here's one 'bonus' of looking like I do. People are extra kind! I get doors opened for me, I was recently at lunch with a dear friend and the waitress kept patting my on the shoulder and telling me to take all the time I needed to figure out what I wanted to order. After I went to the car dealership to see how much I'd get for my old clunker and they were extra careful with me. Not that people aren't in general nice and kind, but it's been stepped up a notch!

I notice I'm mostly more patient too (although my husband might argue that point with some validity!). I hope I retain the appreciation I've found for life and people even after this year is up.

Day Before 5th Chemo

Sep 2, 2010 3:33pm

Tomorrow we have to be at the Mayo for an 8 am blood draw and chemo (if my blood work is ok). Turns out lots of people shifted their chemos to Friday this week in preparation for the holiday so we weren't able to get our nice mid-morning time frame.

The best way to prepare for another few harder days following chemo is to have a fun filled day, so I took all 4 kids to Green Mill for lunch and then Brunswick for a couple of hours of fun playing arcade games.

Round 5 will be done tomorrow by noon!!!

We're too critical of ourselves . . .

Sep 2, 2010 7:57pm

I was talking to a good friend today and she said she wasn't sure how she'd react if she were the one with breast cancer. She thought she'd be feeling sorry for herself a great deal more than I have been. Of course, I know her very well and know full well that's not true at all! She'd be kicking cancer butt because she is one of those women who fight hard for what matters to her and always does the right thing—no matter the consequences. But the conversation reminded me of a question I was pondering shortly before my diagnosis. I read "The Art of Possibility" by Ben Zander and in the book he tells the following story:

In the 1950's two shoe salesmen are sent to Africa to investigate the possibility of their company expanding their business into this continent. When they arrive they each observe that the local population doesn't wear shoes. One salesman telegraphs back:

"We're DOOMED! They don't wear shoes! Am returning home immediately"

The other salesman telegraphs back: "Wonderful business opportunity!! They don't have shoes yet!"

So I had been wondering myself which of the two reactions I usually have when something unexpected happens . . . I thought about it a lot until I got my diagnosis and more of less forgot about the entire thing until my conversation today.

The answer seems to be that we are often the second guy . . . even though we fear we might be the first.

Round 5 Done!

Sep 3, 2010 5:54pm

We had an early chemo appointment today and now I'm done with #5! I also decided to forego the nausea pill they give me alongside the steroids . . . . apparently it might be causing the headaches I get the day after treatment and even though they are manageable, I'd rather not have headaches! The nurses were a bit cautious about me declining the pill but I really haven't had any issues so let's see how this goes. I think the nausea would have kicked in by now and I still feel ok. Fingers crossed!

We also stopped at a greasy spoon before coming home so we could eat lunch (we ordered breakfast though)—maybe that helped too.

I just finished letting the kids color my bald head—they love being able to let loose on Mommy's head. I haven't looked in the mirror yet but did notice Lucy using an awful lot of black . . .

Feeling great!

Sep 4, 2010 6:16pm

No headaches, no nausea and feel great!!!!!!!! We had a busy day running around doing errands and can finally relax now. Saturday is often my "bad day" and it's turning out pretty nice. Plus it's lovely outside and we are going to a Twins game tomorrow—more to look forward to.

Ok—off to grill a juicy steak and stir fry veggies in my new wok. I missed owning a wok!

Take care and enjoy the sun . . .

Decisions, decisions . . .

Sep 5, 2010 11:34am

I'm starting to prepare for a couple of big appointments. I'll actually have to make some sort of intelligent decisions for a change, not just sit there and let people tell me what they are going to do next (which has been nice). I'm meeting both the Radiation Oncologist and the Plastic Surgeon. I'm sure they would tell you they are a team and work together, yadda, yadda, but I like to think of them as the Jekyll and Hyde of surgery. I'm not sure who's Jekyll and who's Hyde though.

The radiation oncologist would rather the plastic surgeon stay away because reconstruction interferes with her work. On the other hand, the plastic surgeon wants to reconstruct immediately after surgery before the radiation oncologist wrecks the skin interfering with his work of art . . .

So I get to arbitrate between these two and come up with how I want things done.

And then I'm sure I'll hear about how the operation can be done, different 'cut lines', etc, etc . . . all EXACTLY what a squeamish person like me wants to discuss and better yet—see pictures of. Yea me!

Now I must say, I've met several women who decided against reconstruction. When you meet someone like that take a close look at her face because you are staring into the face of true inner strength!

As far as I've been told I have all options still available to me ranging from just lumpectomy to the full shebang which I am opting for without looking back. I'm buying that T-shirt that says "Yes, they are fake! My real ones tried to kill me!".

Ahhh . . . the final decision . . . .

Sep 5, 2010 12:12pm

So I was asked by several: what size breasts? Hahaha . . .

I'm practicing saying with a straight face: "So if I go with a double D, does it mean I no longer need to wear a life vest?" or "Is it true I need a face guard for jogging if I go double D?".

But it occurs to me the doctor must have heard every joke in the book and NOT find me very amusing.

Why mess with perfection? I don't want to look any different from what I did before cancer and mastectomies were in my vernacular.

Radiation/Plastic Surgery Appointment

Sep 8, 2010 4:43pm

Yesterday was a real busy day! We met our radiation oncologist who I really liked. Pretty much everyone we come in contact with is caring, professional and very much on their game. She was so clear not only about how plastic surgery can interfere with her duties but also had a fairly good-work around for me. So in short, I wasn't put in a position of needing to weigh pros and cons because she painted a very realistic scenario (that I later was able to deduce the other doctors were aware of and ok with).

After this round of chemo I'll be given a few weeks to recover and then we go to surgery. After surgery I roll right into the second dose of chemo and after that 25 consecutive days of radiation. Apparently radiation really damages the skin, they need to be careful of how much of it hits the heart and lungs (in my case those organs are pretty much in the way) and they also try to get the chest wall lymph nodes just in case. There is no guarantee the radiation oncologist can reach all the places she wants to but there is a strong correlation between receiving radiation and lower rates of recurrence 5 to 10 years down the road. So it'll be worth my skin maybe turning black, the reconstruction being impaired or some of the potential problems that I could encounter 10 years from now.

We then met the plastic surgeon. We were very impressed with him too! State of the art techniques, very principled which is important when choosing a plastic surgeon because I'll know this guy pretty much forever. If there is one doctor I'll be seeing every year for the rest of my life, it's this guy. Good sense of humor and clearly a rock star in his field.

The nice thing is how they are ALL very considerate. They talk about the emotional turmoil of all this just as much as they talk technicalities. Every doctor, every nurse!

Reconstruction could take up to a year so that's pretty much the longest part of it all.

It was nice to have several of them tell me I look good and seem to be doing very well. And one of the nurses tell me I'm very healthy as she looks at my blood work numbers. Always reassuring to hear especially as I notice that as the weeks go by it's a bit harder to bounce back. This past cycle I wasn't quite as tired, but a little tired over a longer period of time.

Of course today I feel awesome chemo-wise! Two more days then I get slammed again . . . hahaha . . . slammed is a bad word to use. I get to receive my 'liquid gold' which is the chemo that is helping me kick butt!

The nurse instructing us on the ins and outs of reconstruction was funny. Very kind, very empathetic but also very interesting. Picture a late 50's woman, lots of make-up, hair colored a deep black, extremely well endowed (perhaps a walking billboard for the latest silicone implant brand) and talks a bit like an infomercial . . . it got a teeny bit uncomfortable at times but amidst the humor, I have to say the lady was so nice, so friendly and very sensitive.

The reconstruction in and of itself is going to be a huge challenge. Another mental battle, I can already tell. I am in awe of all the women out there who have gone through this. Seriously . . . . in awe!

The randomness of it all . . .

Sep 9, 2010 6:57pm

The interesting question as I get to know or hear about all these people who have had cancer: what makes some of us lucky enough to survive and some of us don't? It's not always related to how "far along" the cancer was and it's hopefully not true that some deserve recovery and some less so . . .

Chemo #6

Sep 10, 2010 9:34am

I'm sitting here at the Mayo and my blood work looks good, so we're going ahead with round #6—half way through the first chemo treatment! From now on I start counting down.

It looks like it'll be another beautiful day and I'm really looking forward to the big breakfast I'll have afterwards! We think that helped me have a good week last cycle: chemo followed by huge breakfast . . . who can complain about that?

I been thinking I probably need to start refocusing on "normal" daily activities a little more now that the shock of cancer has subsided. Finding a nice blend of remaining enlightened by it but not taken over by it seems to be important too.

Take care and don't let silly issues get between you and people you care about. We waste so much time sometimes . . .

Final Round #6 Update

Sep 10, 2010 7:19pm

So half way through the chemo drip the trial coordinators came so we can do our weekly exchange of "data". I provide them with my observations of my week with the trial meds (or placebo, we don't know) and they give me a new sheet to fill out. But this time they told me my white blood cells are getting low and the trend suggests would be too low to give me chemo next week unless I get shots to boost their production. Remember how much I hate shots . . .

For the next 6 treatments I will need to get shots every Monday, Tuesday and Wednesday. But it gets worse! The Gods of Irony found this a prime opportunity to have a laugh on me. Get this, I could decide to drive to the Mayo three times a week (not counting Friday!) JUST to spend 30 seconds getting a shot. Well, that makes no sense. Or I could drive to some clinic here and still waste time for a 30 second shot which also makes little sense to me. So the engineer that still lives somewhere inside me made me say to the trial coordinator: "Oh, never mind, I'll give myself the shot at home. It's no problem". Meanwhile my brain is shouting: "Are you NUTS?????? So you're going to stab yourself with a needle 3 times a week for the next 6 weeks??????? That's IT! No more offering up handy dandy solutions for YOU lady!".

So now I have needles in my refrigerator waiting for Monday morning when I get to do this.

And I am sure that when I tell you how THAT adventure goes it'll be funny. Funny for you guys at least . . . .

The shot!

Sep 13, 2010 3:17pm

Today I gave myself my first human growth hormone shot . . .

I was imagining myself sitting on the couch with a syringe glistening in the early morning sun and the sound of sharp metal zinging as I remove the cap and expose it's deadly tip. I envisioned my hand trembling right before the moment when I jab it into my leg and the scene ends with a blood curdling scream heard all around my neighborhood . . .

That, of course, was the most likely scenario for my first shot this morning but fate once again threw me a curveball. Lucy. My 6 year old (who by the way also goes into a complete panic over shots) decided SHE was going to witness the shot and actually strongly suggested she be the one administering it because "I have a Barbie vet kit so I've practiced giving shots to all my toys!!". Err . . . . no.

Additionally I've started my "Lucy, you will need to get a flu shot soon, so be prepared" speech. It's a month long campaign I go through every Fall to convince this child that shots are OK and nothing to be afraid of! So how can I possibly show even a flicker of fear as I stick myself with this thing now?!

So I took her with me to the bathroom, used the little alcohol wipe on my leg, didn't make eye contact with the pointy sharp needle even though Lucy was EXTRAORDINARILY zealous in pointing out just how sharp it looked and how much liquid was inside. I kept remembering the nurse saying "Don't inject it too quickly, it'll sting more . . ."

And now for the anticlimax: I stuck it in, barely felt it, injected the fluid in, barely stung and I was done. Lucy said she was disappointed it didn't bleed at all. I said this proves she shouldn't be afraid of needles because I'm not. I'm so full of it!

My Brave Lucy . . . .

Sep 15, 2010 8:55pm

So I'm getting used to my cancer getting in the way with my family's normal life and frankly feel bad abut that. And today it happened again! I went to take the kids to get their flu shots and Lucy was determined to get the Flu Mist spray in her nose and absolutely NOT the shot. I tried to talk her into the shot because it's more effective than the Mist but for the most part I didn't care and was going to get her the spray version.

I signed both kids in at the clinic, told them I'd give them the Flu Mist and waited for their turn. The nurse came out and the minute she saw me asked politely: "Is anyone in the home immune suppressed?". As in: "Lady you are obviously on chemo but I'm not going to come out an say it . . ."

So the bottom line is that the flu mist is a live virus so I can't be exposed to it. I had to tell Lucy right there in the waiting room that she was going to have to get the shot because otherwise it could make me sick. Surprisingly she just smiled and said "OK, I'll do it then". Wow . . . .

She did cry but she was so brave. I'm so proud of her.

Chemo #7

Posted Sep 17, 2010 3:41pm

After today's treatment I only have 5 more to go . . . I'm starting to count down. And between now and my last treatment we are all going to Florida on vacation for some sun and beach action. I can't wait! I do envision some adventures trying to take 4 young kids on a plane however . . .

I was also seen by the oncologist for a check today and the good news is they are no longer able to find the tumor! Take that! Cancer messed with the wrong chick!

Strength and Vulnerability

Sep 18, 2010 10:25pm

A dear friend and I were talking about how a cancer diagnosis is hard on pretty much everyone involved and we all deal with it differently. It's largely why I see this battle as belonging to all of you as much as it belongs to me.

It seems as though we all alternate between being strong and being vulnerable through this. I think the key is that we tend to take turns on who is feeling strong and who is feeling vulnerable. But I've become very aware of how virtually all of you have gone through some degree of personal struggle as you also contemplate illness, life and the inevitable fear that it all evokes. I'll be strong for you and you'll be strong for me. You get to tell me how this has felt for you and I get to tell you on a regular basis what I'm thinking—that makes me lucky. The beauty of it all is that no storm lasts forever and this too shall pass. Because it will!

I've learnt to come to terms with the vulnerable moments and tried to stop calling them weakness. It's becoming more and more obvious to me that being vulnerable and being strong are not on opposite sides of a scale. It's all part of the whole we are as people. A good cry followed by the knowledge that we can overcome anything is now perfectly normal. It's more like those are sister emotions are not in conflict. I think I was very black and white regarding the human condition. Black and white, and wrong! Accepting all emotions without letting them completely take over seems to work well. Acceptance really is a powerful gift. A very powerful gift. We're often so unhappy about so many things about ourselves and it's such a shame we are so critical. I see it everyday with people I care about and wish they (and I) were a bit softer. Like they say: there is no way to happiness, happiness is the way. And there's plenty of reason to just be happy, even through the occasional tears.

It's gonna be a good day

Sep 22, 2010 8:24am

I couldn't wait to get up this morning! Ok, so maybe part of it was having my two year olds foot on my head and my 6 year olds legs across my back and my husband stole the covers but still . . . . I feel AWESOME today! I know it takes weeks to recover from chemo (I'm told it can take up to a year and not everything will be the same) but it still feels SO good to come out of the cycle low point and start to feel like a normal person again.

And to top it all off: the sun is coming up and looks like another beautiful day. How lucky is that?!

Bonfire of Vanities . . . . literally

Sep 23, 2010 2:56pm

Had I been asked 6 months ago if I considered myself vain, I'd have said no without missing a beat. I never really spent anytime at all thinking about my hairstyle, never paid a lot of attention to the latest fashion or dedicated more than 30 seconds to how moisturized my skin was. And I don't think there are a lot of people out there who would say that who we are is all about how we look. It's about who you are inside, how you treat others, yadda, yadda, yadda . . . . Right?

So suddenly faced with losing my hair, having chemo wreck my skin, being left with what could be some size-able scaring and sticking out like a sore thumb wherever I go (yea, I get stared at a lot) was disconcerting. So I wasn't terribly proud of the fact that my looks changing was bothering me when it first started. I wanted to say: "My hair is going to fall out? Oh, I don't care! I'm more than just my hair you know. I'm a myself regardless of my hair and regardless of whether I'll be left with scars. Nope, it doesn't bother me in the slightest because I know better!".

But time passes and hair falls out (or gets shaven and insists on growing back but that's a different story), skin changes with chemo and I learn more about the possible impact of surgery and radiation . . . . and somehow I forget about how I used to look. And somehow I still feel the same. Well . . . . actually I don't feel the same. I feel more like me than I did when all the other stuff was in the way. How odd is that? I'm more Joana than I was when I let vanities dictate—even to a small extent—how I saw myself. And it doesn't seem to make a lick of difference in how the people I care about interact with me.

Now I walk around and catch myself surprised when people stare or ask if I'm alright because I often completely forget that I don't look "normal".

So I say, burn all vanities and let the real you out!

Time warp . . . .

Sep 24, 2010 10:15am

I've said this numerous times, the Mayo doesn't feel like a hospital; it feels like a warm place you go to get healed. I love it here. It really feels like going home to your grandma's house and you know she'll cook your favorite meal. And guess what else feels like your grandma's house? The waiting rooms. It's like you enter this time warp and you're living back in the 1940's! It's not the decor that I'm sure is perfectly neutral and timeless; it's the overall ambiance. If you find a nice comfy recliner (yes, they have recliners in the waiting rooms) and observe you'll see for the most part couples in their 60's and 70's. I immediately picture them as a young couple sometime during the war; those old black and white photos of a smiling woman with her sailor fiancee . . . It's hard to ignore the large flowery print on the lady's blouse and the white shoes and white socks the men favor. I think there must be some senior citizen discount on those things . . . either that or some bizarre statistical anomaly is going on because 100% of the men over 50 appear to have chosen that today (come to think of it—every day). Oh, and then the constant muzak. I've been keeping track of the muzak. They favor the 1936 "For Sentimental Reasons", Bing Crosby tunes, a variety of orchestra renditions of Beverly Sisters hits and of course old Blue Eyes. I noticed they don't play "My Way" and have to chuckle as I imagine the meeting where someone says "We can't play 'My Way'. It's going to disturb the patients". I don't think it'd upset anyone nearly as much as just the mere presence of this incessant muzak! I swear it can drive a perfectly calm person to drink.

I think I'm going to suggest they change it up a little. We've done the 40's and 50's for at least two months now according to my tracking, so I think we should go disco 70's. Bee Gees, Barry Manilow, Billy Joel and Captain and Tennille. If I'm going to go slowly crazy, let's at least make it quick . . .

After today: 4 more treatments to go!

The Dreaded Conversation . . .

Sep 24, 2010 11:24pm

I just had to have the hardest conversation with Lucy . . .

At night, it's part of our bedtime routine that I sit between their beds and hold hands with both Lucy and Daniel and we talk quietly for about 5 minutes. I've always wanted to have some time when all is still and I can gage their real feelings about random things and they have a safe place to tell me what is on their minds. There are too many sad stories of parents for whom tragedy strikes with their teens and they felt they never saw it coming . . . I really want to prevent that if I can. Hopefully my kids will know they can talk to me and some of that might remain when they are suddenly smart teens and I am just a dumb mom.

My cancer came up for Lucy and I will try to reproduce the conversation we had.

"Mommy, how many more times do you have to get medicine?"

"Only 4 more times and then I get to take a break for 4 weeks!! Then I do surgery which means they take out the spot where cancer was growing just to be extra safe. After that I take even more medicine and by the time you are done with 1st grade, I will have beaten this cancer and be all done with this! Neat, huh??"

"Yea . . . what do you mean beat cancer?"

"I mean cancer is like a monster that I am fighting and I am going to win! I am already winning. Remember I told you the doctor said he could not find it in me anymore?"

"Yea . . . so what are you fighting? What is cancer fighting for?"

At this point I know what she is getting at. She knows perfectly well that her grandfather died of melanoma and that her friends' sister died of cancer last year. I sense she wants me to say it out loud. I still don't have the courage to flat out say it, so I reply:

"Cancer wants to grow in other parts of my body and make me sick"

"And then what happens after you get sick?" She insists . . .

"Well . . . . I would get very very sick and at some point . . . well . . . die"

She just lies there holding my hand and looking at me blinking. I have a rule when parenting. NEVER make a promise you don't intend to keep. Never. But right then and there I decide to amend my rule. Only make a promise you have GOOD CONFIDENCE you will keep. I debate this internally for a few agonizing seconds but I tell her:

"Lucy, I am NOT going to die ok? I am already winning the fight and I WILL be ok. I will take all the medicine I can to be extra sure; and the medicine will make me tired but that's all. Remember we talk about being stubborn and how sometimes it's bad and sometimes it's good? And that, like you, I am also stubborn sometimes? Well, it's good I am stubborn because it means I am GOING to be just fine"

She seems to accept this and doesn't seem outwardly disturbed. She never really has seemed at all upset by all this and I think tends to tell me her thoughts.

And out of the blue we hear: "I wanna say somink! I wanna talk about my birfday!" Daniel was feeling left out . . . hehehe.

I leave the kids to sleep and when I return 10 minutes later to check on them they are both sleeping like angels.

I think I'm going to cry myself to sleep. I never wanted to have to tell my children that I could die. Not when they are so young and need me so much.

Hats off to sick people!

Sep 26, 2010 5:46pm

There is something very isolating about being the sick one. I really admire people who live with chronic conditions and who manage pain and illness on a daily basis. The effort to just be "normal" is huge and really wears one down. I can honestly say I don't remember what it feels like to not be in some sort of pain or hard to ignore discomfort. I really dont remember feeling healthy anymore and its tiring and oddly isolating from the rest of the world. But at the same time I think of all the people who just got a cancer diagnosis and who are about to start down this long path . . . or those who have been fighting for years and years. Wow . . .

Thankfully today hasn't turned out to be a very hard day. I think most of my other cycles had me struggling more by Sunday than this time.

I can't wait for the day when I just don't feel ill anymore. I hope I won't take that feeling for granted because I sure used to.

Back on track . . .

Sep 27, 2010 3:09pm

After a couple of mentally challenging days I am feeling a lot better! I'm lucky enough to have a husband who helps me put things into perspective and remember what's important during those moments when I'm just exhausted of all the treatments, fed up of feeling sick and feeling overwhelmed with the long recovery path still ahead. There's a reason they say that being the caregiver is harder than being the sick person . . .

I am definitely not good at letting myself be sick and not feel well. Maybe instead of fighting it, I should just embrace the days that are crappy. Maybe I'd be more patient and tolerant of the chemo side effects if I was afraid this cancer was going to kill me, but I genuinely don't believe it has what it takes to bring me down :o)

It's nice to hear that the drug combo I'm on now is the worst of it. My doctors have told me the same so it can only get better after October 25th—my last AC chemo treatment! And to be honest, I've reacted extremely well to it all, I've been lucky. I hear of much harder reactions from other people out there (and from the trial coordinators at the Mayo). The second chemo round should be easier and radiation should be fairly easy according to my radiation oncologist.

My goal for the next few days: to get myself back to a mental state where I am at peace with the treatments I still need to go through. I don't want to just "push through" them because that catches up to you too . . . it takes energy to muscle through anything. Ideally I can return to living in the moment and just be happy because I have tons of reasons to be.

Sleeping Woes

Sep 30, 2010 11:47am

One funny thing with chemo is the list of symptoms . . . first of all they are endless and no one really gives you the entire list. And second, the list is comprised of a series of antitheses. Constipation or diarrhea, sleepiness or sleeplessness and on and on . . .

After the first number of weeks I was certain that sleeping was going to be one of my things. I slept deeply most nights, except when kids would wake me up. Not bad, seemed normal to me. But lately I've swung over to the sleepless nights side, much to my frustration. I can't fall asleep nor can I stay asleep for more than an hour at a time. I can't get comfortable no matter what I try. Last night I pictured Sleeping Beauty who is lucky enough to get a 100 year nap—right around the amount of sleep I'd like to get right now too!

I think part of it is the stupid mattress and Saturday we'll go buy a new one. But part of me wonders if it's also chemo related and no matter how nice a mattress we purchase, I might need to deal with being awake. At least I'll be on a cushier bed!

(I just occurred to me that likening myself to Sleeping Beauty doesn't really work. I'm bald and wear cotton hats in bed . . . . I think I look a lot more like Dopey of the Seven Dwarves . . . .)

Chemo#9 underway!!!!

Oct 1, 2010 1:53pm

After today: 3 treatments to go! Yea! I'm starting to see the light at the end of this tunnel as I discuss the timing of my surgery appointment with the trial coordinator. I'll be done with both clinical trials after my 12 chemos: the new chemo drug trial and the new imaging technique. I'm very curious to do that last imaging session to see if they can pick up any cancer cells. My surgeon had told us that reaching the end of chemo with no tumor left is "the perfect world" so I'm happy that's where I'm at. But the new imaging should be able to detect miniscule cancer regions, so let's see what it shows us.

By mid November I'll have a surgery plan in place and I'm on to the next adventure. I'm sure I'll be a wreck over the prospect of being "put under" for the surgery. I'd much rather they give me some massive spinal block but leave me awake to supervise and provide direction as they do surgery. I'd want to literally be a talking head, numb from the neck down and obnoxious from the neck up.

My good mood has returned. Somehow it's become clear that I'm in full control of how I am feeling independently of the situations or the people around me. It's virtually impossible to be trapped in hopelessness . . . . what an interesting and comforting feeling.

I hope you have a wonderful day. Take a second to feel happy and think of one thing to be thankful for . . . . do it right now. C'mon! You got a second.

Cooking and Photos

Oct 3, 2010 12:36pm

Even though I'm feeling pretty tired from the chemo and very low red blood cell counts I'm so pleased I have found the energy to start cooking! One of my favorite things to do is cook a big meal; something I don't always have time to do with all the kids running around and the insanity of weekday activities. But I have a big fat whole chicken in the slow cooker and let's see how it turns out in 6 hours. Lots of olive oil, garlic and my own mix of spices rubbed all over it and underneath the skin. It's going to be awesome!

Then I made some banana bread—one of the kids favorites. Daniel is the most passionate about banana bread which he calls 'cake'.

Later today I'm going to try to go through some photos and get them in albums. I love taking photos, we have a lot of them framed around the house but mostly I have them digitalized. I have been meaning to make a physical photo album for each kid. Something I can give them someday when they grow up.

My two favorite things! Food and photos.

When you just have to ask for help . . .

Oct 4, 2010 3:39pm

It's been one of the rougher days symptom wise where nausea has really been dogging me, my body hurts and my eyesight is not reliable no matter how much water I drink to stay hydrated. I kept Daniel home today because he had pinkeye and I was planning on taking him to the doctor but at some point realized I can't drive him. It's just not safe when my eyes act like they are today—my vision is terrible. Additionally I want to go on a field trip with Lucy and her class tomorrow. The whole day outside at the Arboretum. I'm a little concerned I wont be able to manage a full day outside, Lucy's girl scouts followed by gymnastics.

So I bit the bullet and asked for help in a way that I really don't like to . . . help in taking care of my kids which is always hard to give up!

Daniel's dad came to pick him up and take him to urgent care for me and he'll end up keeping the kids tonight too so I can rest. I know he is more than happy to take the kids but it's so hard to give them up. I love spending as much time as I can with them and watching Daniel cry because he wants to stay home with me is so painful. He asked me if after his dad took him to the doctor he could come back to my house and I had to tell him no which made him cry. I feel awful. He's at that age where it's all about Mom, so it's harder for him to leave.

I know this is one point in time but I hate that cancer takes away time with my children. I'm mad cancer takes so much away all the time. When I'm done with this, I'm going to make sure I do whatever I can to not let cancer do this to other people.

Barnacles!

Oct 5, 2010 11:48am

I was going to take Lucy on her field trip today—we were both pretty excited about it! But I woke up and realized I can't stand up for long without feeling faint, my heart palpates and my vision is just terrible. I called the Mayo and they instructed me to either drive right down to the Mayo NOW or head to a local emergency room NOW.

Obviously I couldn't take Lucy on her field trip which is disappointing beyond belief! Steve will take me to the ER in a little bit; we'll bring Daniel along too for what might be a long day. I think this might involve fluids and maybe a blood transfusion . . .

I'll keep you posted but my guess is it'll be some uneventful boring stay at the ER causing me to also miss Lucy's gymnastics! I suspect I need to eat more red meat . . .

Physically I'll be just fine. Emotionally I am so irritated by this!!!!!! &*^$&%$#!#!!!!!!!!!

Much much better!

Oct 5, 2010 8:17pm

So I guess I'm supposed to drink a TON of fluids and eat red meat for 3 weeks . . .

We went the the ER and set up camp. You literally need to set up a camp when you have a 2 year old with zero attention span and a husband who really needs to get some work done and is getting very proficient at working in hospitals.

We had a couple of kid books, a toy Thomas the Tank and my work laptop playing 1940's Mickey episodes to keep Daniel busy. He was his usual charming self with the nurses and doctor :o)

I'm amazed by how cautiously I'm treated because I'm a chemo patient. I just can't get over that . . . they rush me into triage, immediately find me a room (and I think bump me ahead of people in line) when the truth is all I was is dizzy and weak. All my blood work showed me with low counts on everything but just your run of the mill chemo stuff, no serious anemia and thankfully no need for a transfusion. I was dreading a blood transfusion . . . somehow it freaks me out to think of people pumping blood into me. They gave me a liter of fluid and about 30 minutes after leaving the ER I felt awesome!

The Mayo called me back too—they are watching me like a hawk. Essentially telling me it must be fluids and somewhat low red blood cells so I'm ordered to drink like a fish and eat red meat.

Meanwhile Lucy was so gracious about my not going on the trip and we are now planning a girls only afternoon. She's becoming so understanding, so tolerant . . . I don't like appearing weak in front of my kids so letting her see me needing to sit down and tell her I couldn't make it was hard. But I know there is little point hiding life from either of them. Life has taught me that nothing is permanent, everything changes and junk happens. My gift to my kids is to teach them how to handle the blessings with thankfulness and the problems with grace and kindness.

Thanks for all your thoughts and concern! I'm a tough cookie and if cancer isn't going to get me; a little dizziness won't phase me :o)

Communication is hard . . . .

Oct 7, 2010 9:21am

Something yesterday reminded me of this conversation I had this year with a Senior General Mills VP I ran into in the hall, a few days after I got my promotion.

VP: "Hi Joana! I hear congratulations are in order!"

J: "Oh, thanks, yes. I was flattered"

VP: "I was surprised I didn't know until now . . . . You didn't come tell me!"

J: "Well, I didn't know until it was final either I guess . . . ."

So I'm thinking first of all this guy would probably know whether or not a promotion was coming down the line for me months before I'd ever find out, so him not knowing about it seemed odd. And even odder he expected me to call him with the news? Seriously?! He's a busy guy; I'm not going to bother him with my little promotion news . . . plus it feels like boasting and my mother told me to never boast.

VP: "So are you happy?"

J: "Oh yes, of course. Not that I need it, I just like to be able to do what I enjoy"

You get the gist of it, right? We both part ways and I head off to the cafeteria confused. Well . . . turns out he was NOT talking about my promotion but about the fact I had gotten MARRIED a few months earlier!!!!!!

My guess is he walked right to HR, pulled out my file and had them check the IDIOT box.

I had a similar albeit less career limiting conversation yesterday with my oncologist. I usually talk to oncology nurses and the clinical trial coordinators and rarely to my oncologist directly. There's been no need. But he called me yesterday after I told them I was still feeling some odd stuff in my chest. I really like my oncologist, Dr. Sideras. Picture Al Pacino in one of those subdued quiet roles. Awfully serious, actually very caring but you get the sense that if he yells at you, you'll feel the size of a pea. He gives me a sense of confidence and I trust him. Plus, he humors me when I want to get treatments done sooner rather than later . . .

I'm on the phone with him talking about my symptoms for a good 10 minutes. I expected him to tell me to drink even more, or tell me they might reduce the amount of chemo drugs because he had told me previously these drugs negatively impact the heart. I felt fine, just some mild stuff going on, but I was flattered he took the time to call me . . . . until he finally said: "Ok . . . I think we can probably rule out heart attack unless this persists after you take ibuprofen for a few hours". WHAT???!?!?!?!?!?! We've been talking to see if I'm having a HEART ATTACK????? Are you kidding me????????

Obviously I'm not having a heart attack, I'm perfectly fine (although I do have an EKG and chest x-ray suddenly scheduled for Friday). I'm sure it's all just fine, I feel great, lots of energy after my ER visit and very happy the sun is out. I'm glad they are careful at the Mayo, but good grief people! I'm NOT having a heart attack!

(Life Lesson: always ask what the conversation is about)

Getting there . . . .

Oct 8, 2010 4:34pm

Chemo #10—2 more to go after a 10 day break!

Today has been a busy day! Blood test, chest x-ray, EKG, oncology check and now chemo to finish up the day.

The good news is my chest and heart seem just fine and the great news (but not surprising, just nice to keep hearing) is that the oncologist still can't find the tumor! Not that it would have disappeared 3 weeks ago and reappeared now, but still . . . I like to keep hearing it's gone.

We are trying to think of any possible thing we might need during our Florida vacation particularly any medicines I might need. We won't have car down there since the goal is to sit on the beach and the very last thing I want to do is have to go to a doctor or a pharmacy during those 5 days!

Sigh . . . . these chemo drugs start working right away. I've been sitting here for 15 minutes and I already feel the effects. Ick.

Home stretch!

Weekend activity

Oct 9, 2010 11:31am

Going apple and pumpkin picking today . . . . we need to bleed off all this kid energy! Daniel thinks I'm a jungle gym but I already feel like I got hit by a truck. Wait, no. A fleet of trucks :o)

Beautiful day out again though. Isn't it wonderful when the sun is out in the morning?

Almost vacation . . . .

Oct 12, 2010 9:55am

I'm really looking forward to tomorrow although I'm a tiny bit apprehensive about how much energy I'll have for a full day of travel to Florida. But it's going to be fun to take the kids on this adventure—the flight will be one of the highlights of the trip for them so I can't wait to see their faces.

As the chemo cycles slowly come to an end my mind is starting to look to the second cycle of chemo that's coming after surgery and frankly getting anxious over that. These are the types of thoughts that trip us up in life . . . . looking ahead and getting anxious over what is yet to come; might come; could come; etc . . . . a waste of time and energy but a pattern we all fall prey to.

No matter what we are going through, it's been critical for me to focus exclusively on what is going on at the present time. And not just to keep anxiety and worry at bay, but there is so much going on at the present moment that I'd miss if I were only paying attention to some fictitious future I've made up in my brain. I'd miss out on noticing the humanity of those around me, I'd miss out on deepening my relationships with those I care about and I'd miss out on the moments when I feel great and so fortunate when my energy starts coming back. So I'm working hard to stay focused because after 10 weeks of constant chemo. Perhaps my oncologist will decide to do a short second chemo round, or even none at all! But until I find that out—i have a fun trip ahead, a few weeks without meds in November which will be a huge blessing and I get closer to the cure.

I think of those miners in Chile—trapped underground for as long as I've been doing chemo. I get to breathe fresh air, I get to be with my family and friends, I get to fly to Florida. Talk about a mental and physical challenge with those 33 men . . . . I'd best start REALLY appreciating how lucky I am right now! Seriously . . . .

Surgery scheduled for November 19th!!!

Oct 15, 2010 7:51pm

I used to watch these interviews on TV of people going through these life changing ordeals like say, oh for arguments sake, breast cancer and they sit in the interview chair with a wise serene expression saying wise insightful things. And I used to think that's how they went through their entire journey: wise, serene and insightful. So my immediate thought would be "My gosh, there is no way I'd be so strong and graceful if something like that happened to me!" And of course immediately feel bad about myself. We see these snapshots of people going through strife and assume it's how the entire thing proceeds for them.

Well, now I know that's not really true. It's true the hardship changes you. It's true that you become wiser, more serene and insightful. It's true the journey is a blessing in disguise and you transform into someone richer and with more to offer others and frankly yourself.

But there is a decent amount of time when it's less attractive. No one really tells you about those times . . . the times when you wish it was over, the times you are angry this will never let you go even after remission, the times your emotions are so raw you barely recognize yourself anymore. We prefer to only share the moments that make us look heroic, it's human nature.

This so called journey doesn't really have an end (because it doesn't end in remission, it never ends). Regardless, this so called journey is the best thing that ever sucked that is happening to me.

But a word to the wise: don't be fooled into thinking that strong wise serene person is like that the entire time. None of us are and guess what? It's ok.

Last day of vacation . . . .

Oct 16, 2010 3:31pm

I'll send a longer update once I get back—too many adventures to tell—but it's been awesome! Beautiful beaches, hot weather, kids having fun, my energy level is higher than normal (although my mouth still tastes odd) and tomorrow we go the airport at 5 am . . . 5 am!!! How we get 4 kids up and ready by then escapes me . . .

I posted a couple of pics but took hundreds :o)

Chemo #11 after vacation

Oct 18, 2010 8:30pm

The best surprise about our vacation on Sanibel Island was my energy level. For the most part I felt pretty normal; just a little tired but nothing that impacted how busy we were! It was awesome!!!!! I forgot all about my cancer for a lot of the time :o) How cool was that?! I even boogie boarded one afternoon. For the most part I had some good thoughts about how we all go through this process but for the most part I really felt as though that part of my life had been left behind except for a few moments.

I grew up close to the ocean and being close to it again was wonderful.

The kids loved the whole experience from flight to ocean to seeing dolphins up close . . . so fun.

Returning home was sad. I'm starting to plan our net trip already!

Today I completed my 11th chemo and we are planning for surgery on the 19th of November. One more and then I start focusing on recovering from it and getting ready for my operation and healing from that. I don't know what comes after surgery and my guess is nothing will get set in stone until surgery is done and they see what's in there. They literally test all tissue for cancer cells as the surgery is proceeding so they'll learn a lot during those hours.

Almost done with this part of recovery! Yea!!!!!!!!!!!!!!! I'm in an awesome mood today ;o) How about you?

One more week . . .

Oct 21, 2010 10:32am

It's almost hard to believe that a week from today I'll be coming out of a chemo cycle WITHOUT a new one coming on it's heels. It's almost hard to believe . . . I've gotten so used to going through this that I'm not sure I remember not feeling either weak or nauseous or just plain exhausted. I know with surgery it'll be a new set of physical and mental challenges but I doubt it'll be anything like this chemo marathon.

I'm really looking forward to being done!!!!!! I never want to look at another nausea pill again!

Another advantage of starting to feel normal will be seeing friends again. The best medicine is just chatting and laughing with people . . . turns out I'm an extrovert; go figure!

Girls Day Out

Oct 22, 2010 11:51am

Today Lucy and I are going to have an all girls day out. We watched a movie already, are planning on going to paint ceramics for a while followed by lunch at her favorite restaurant (Applebees, of course) and then a bit of shopping.

I posted a couple of photos we took this morning already—note the missing tooth!

In the evening I'm taking Steve out somewhere nice. He deserves a break!

Take care and enjoy the day!

. . . . I forget

Oct 24, 2010 12:33pm

I don't do details. I really really don't. For those of you that know me well, you know that I only mildly acknowledge the existence of due process for things and details around events and you also know I am not going to be the person you come to for any sort of assistance in those matters. I came to terms with that in my twenties working on my doctorate. I was supposed to care about the nitty gritty stuff, I was supposed to write my thesis as if it were to be evaluated by the pound and I was supposed to be ecstatic over every split hair . . . yet I wasn't and came to accept it. It's true I'm still a geek at heart, I get all excited over episodes of NOVA, really truly miss my Statistics classes and love it when people show my their data. But my brain never really gravitated naturally towards caring about it for long periods of time. It's people that truly fascinate me. People are amazingly complicated beautiful universes all contained in one body. (There is at least one of you out there who is throwing up in his mouth a little bit right now. And you know who you are!!!! ;o).

For someone who thrives on being around people starting my post college life working on a thesis in a University was probably not playing to my strengths although I confess I did enjoy every second of it. And if additionally one decides to work with a deadly form of a bacteria, it's no surprise there were few fellow research students looking to share a lab with me . . . my own advisor kept his distance in case of contamination! Geez . . . Chicken.

So I have plenty of evidence that I am a people person, prefer to think in terms of relationships and not in terms of facts; just ask my husband. I'm telling you all this as a way to excuse, pardon, explain, my total and complete breakdown when it comes to remembering ANYTHING lately. If you want me to recall ANYTHING, just know I'll say "I don't know". "What was breakfast?". I don't remember. "When is your next appointment at the Mayo?" Aside from Monday I have no idea even though I just looked at my very full schedule pre-surgery. "Have you paid our bills?" Our what . . . ?

I could blame chemo but I'm choosing to say it's just because I'm a free spirit who it wonderfully focused on other things. I just don't remember what . . .

Hot, hot, hot

Oct 25, 2010 11:08am

Ode to the hot flash

Before my life was so simple
Always cold, so turn up the heat
But now my body's gone crazy
And drumming to a different beat
I'll be feeling my normal self
Warm house and baths, my soft spot
But suddenly out of the blue
My collar begins to feel hot
It starts hot and very flush
Progresses to a fiery attack
I feel a volcano inside me
You could fry a few eggs on my back
As it came, it leaves with a force
From blaring AC back to my flannel
Steve finds it funny of course:
"What demon did you just channel??"

I'm waiting for my blood work to come back so we can get my last chemo treatment (for now) underway followed by 2 different breast imaging to close out the 2 clinical trials I'm a part of and as information for the surgeons. I'll likely have more chemo after although my oncologist hasn't told me what his plan is yet; he'll wait to see what they find at surgery. But my type of cancer is a rarer type of breast cancer and known to be aggressive so my guess is they err on the side of caution.

I'll miss the trial coordinators though. So many wonderful kind people keeping an eye on me these past 12 weeks. They'll follow my progress for years to come and still meet with me on a regular basis but certainly not as often. At the same time, I'm going to be glad to know this is the last time I need to go through the tough weekly recovery from the Abraxane and Carboplatin—two of the ickier chemo drugs out there. I'm hoping whatever I get for my second round is an "easier" drug to manage. I've been lead to believe that's probably the case, so one can only hope!! :o)

I'm SO thankful for all that's happened. I really am! Cancer, chemo and chemically induced menopause but it's clearer to me than it ever was that I'm so fortunate and there is so much worse out there. The kids are great, smiling is an easy choice to make everyday, since we are what we think we have full control over THAT even if little control over everything else, people are wonderful and rise to the occasion every time and we're all here for each other.

Make sure to find the time to do or say one kind thing today. Then pat yourself on the back for it

Life

Oct 31, 2010 2:04pm

I've said this several times, you get cancer and you start looking at your life drastically differently. There is really nothing like it. I used to think I was very introspective and appreciative of my family, my kids, my good fortune at work . . . but it's really not quite the same as when cancer strikes. It also makes every single experience you have be amplified by 100 and your thoughts about every event that much stronger. I know it's unpopular for someone with cancer to talk about their own death because it sounds as though they are giving up. Well, let me be clear on this point: I don't even like to say I am "fighting" cancer because I'm not. I have BEATEN cancer and am just going through these small details like surgery and some added treatments but the fact is it's been beaten already so I'm not going to waste time thinking that the battle is still on. Nevertheless, this experience has made me closer to my mortality and how short life really can be. Given that, who should we be in this life? What kind of wife, what kind of mother and what kind of friend . . . and how do all those things interact together.

It seems as though everywhere I look there is miscommunication between people. I don't think I know anyone who doesn't have some sort of issues with a relationship in their lives. I sit here and try to think of one person I know who doesn't have some story. And it's never something we can just brush off, right? Relationships, other people, matter. It's amazing how central to our survival positive loving relationships are, yet we are all so inadequate at them a lot of the times.

Many wise people out there have cracked the code of why and I think they are right. For whatever reason we as humans have decided two things: it's crucial to be "right" and it's crucial to keep our pride intact. Additionally we are for the most part terrible listeners so all those human "virtues" put together make us terrible relationship nurturers. The one thing scientifically proven to be required for children to grow up healthy, the one thing we are so dependent on to survive.

Who teaches us to protect our pride at all cost? Who teaches us that being alone and right is more important than the other persons feelings? Why are we so busy thinking of an answer instead of truly listening to what other people are trying to tell us even if it's something we don't want to hear? I'm putting working on this at the top of my list of things to do and it needs to remain there until it's fully accomplished . . . might take a few decades but worth the effort, don't you think?

Enjoying the upswing

Nov 4, 2010 10:56pm

It's been over a week without chemo and I'm really feeling a lot better. I have to confess I'm still pretty tired and reach the end of the day exhausted, my muscles hurt when I walk up stairs and I'm still nauseous often but I'm determined to not let this get in the way of me having full days. I've decided I really need some fun, busy days before I get tied down again as I recover from my surgery.

Our kids . . .

Nov 9, 2010 10:33am

Tomorrow we go back down to the Mayo Clinic for a series of appointments. I haven't been there since October 25th, my last chemo of this first chemo round, and it feels like years! I'm not necessarily looking forward to going back although I never looked at the Mayo as a hospital. They have it set up with an ambiance that really feels more like a beautiful mall or monument. It's a safe warm place, not a cold scary medical facility. At the same time I think I am ready to move to the next step and deal with the surgery. I'm not in a hurry and will fully enjoy the next 10 days, but I'm also not dreading it. I'm finally ready to go ahead with it and am actually looking forward to getting it underway.

I've had a lot of time to think about family and parenthood as I try to get my body recovered from the chemo and ready for the 19th. If you look back at your life, at what you thought your life was going to be like when you were 20 years old and where you are now, it was probably different. Chances are, your life took a bunch of different twists and turns, some good and some challenging but nevertheless I doubt your life was a straight line from point A to point B. I know mine wasn't! I think we all acknowledge those different experiences made us richer and wiser, better parents, better spouses and better friends. So a good thing, right? We don't want life to be a merry-go-round if it can be a roller coast, especially if we only get something like 80 years on this planet. Who wants beige when you can have multi-colored?

So why is it that I can recognize and celebrate the richness and messiness of life but when it comes to my kids, I want perfect (when I say perfect, read "boring"). We want our kids to go through their lives with no difficulties, everything has to happen at the right time, they need to go through school with no issues (and above average!), they need to find the right college major the day they register and pass all classes. They shouldn't have relationship difficulties with anyone, get married first and have their own kids about 2.5 years later . . . . and when things don't go like this we worry our kids are doomed! Doomed!! I feel like Lucy is doomed when she has some strife with another little kid in her class. Daniel is doomed because lately he refuses to talk and seems to think it's funny to just grunt. And then I proceed to give myself the hardest time because of all these things and I see a lot of my friends with kids go through the same type of emotions.

Think of someone you look up to and admire. Someone who makes you want to be a better person. I'd be willing to bet the person you're thinking of didn't have the type of life we obsess over our kids having. The squeaky clean, easy, boring life . . . . Do we seriously want our kids lives to be beige? Sometimes I act like I do!

How quickly they change . . .

Nov 9, 2010 2:59pm

So I had mentioned Daniel has decided he wont speak anymore. He has pretty much not said a word other than grunting and pointing since Sunday . . .

Well today I told him we were going to the store and after we'd go out and enjoy the warm weather by going to the park. He looked at me. Blinked. Frowned. And then said: "I going to talk to you now. I going to say words now mommy. I DONT WANT GO TO STORE! I MAD AT YOU!" Of course it didn't end there. For the next 2 hours he didn't stop talking going from "I not happy, I mad. I mad at my sucker, I mad and car because car not going to playground and I want go to playground, I not want go to big kid playground, I want go to little boy playground; I little boy" to then deciding he was super buddies with the lady checking us out of Target and saying "I buy Mickey diapers. I get big boy diapers but I don't want diaper change, I don't have poopy, I don't need diaper change, I make poopy go away all by myself so no change!". And on and on . . . . and on.

Now we're back home after running our errands and playing at the little boy playground and he still won't stop talking. It's this non stop string of things he has to say. He's making up for not wanting to say a word to me (or anyone) for days! Holy moly! I can hardly get a word in edgewise here . . . . "Mommy, I go play on your phone and I go watch Thomas on TV. You put it on for me. You go get water, I thirsty and you go get cup for me. I like drink water Mommy, I like your water" (It's not really MY water, it's the city of Lakeville water but I'll take credit).

I have to go . . . I just heard a voice say "I don't need diaper change Mommy!!!". We all know what that means . . .

Day back at Mayo

Nov 10, 2010 9:14pm

Whew, what a long day at the Mayo today! We went in for several appointments starting with me giving blood samples for the clinical trial. It's probably the last time they see me until after my whole treatment is done and then they follow me every 6 months. It's always disconcerting to see all the vials they need to fill! It's like they are taking a few gallons of blood! Ick! After that I had to go see the eye doctor because of all the issues I was having and it turns out my eyesight is perfect (docs words, not mine ;o). The theory is that the nausea pills, the fatigue, the dehydration and other factors they don't yet understand about chemo drugs were really affecting my eye sight and it should go back to normal at some point. My last appointment was with my oncologist and he was running SO late. He's really good and clearly always very busy, so I wasn't surprised when an hour passed and we were still waiting. The bottom line is regardless of what they find in surgery—still some cancer left or if it's all gone—I am going ahead with 4 more chemo treatments (Adriamycin every 2 weeks). Given my age and the type of cancer it's just wiser to go full throttle with treatments and not skip anything. I'm not doing more than most breast cancer patients do, this is all standard treatment but the question did arise given how well I responded to this first chemo set. I know it's going to be hard to go back to chemotherapy but I can certainly deal with a few more weeks if I need to just to make sure this I kill this thing for good!

My focus now needs to be getting ready for surgery and making sure I only spend one night in the hospital. Lucy has a school event she is very excited about on the 22nd and I NEED to be well enough to make it there. The key will be for me to start moving as soon as possible and making sure I keep pain under control to speed up healing. It'll all work out, I'm sure.

Weekends

Nov 13, 2010 10:03pm

I've been really trying to have some fun these past couple of weekends. Last weekend we had fun with my stepsons and this weekend it's Lucy and Daniel. It's not as though I'm going off to war, it's just a surgery that lots of women go through and recover from after a few weeks but nevertheless I've wanted to enjoy the kids before I have to tell them to not bump into me or to be gentle around me. Today was hilarious! Daniel went through another bout of non-stop talking before going back to grunting. Lucy had her friend Addison over to play and when those two get together it's the cutest thing. They both put on a concert for me and it was so hard to keep a straight face through it. They sang "Yellow Submarine" but somehow kept getting stuck in some musical twilight zone loop and kept repeating the chorus and even that wasn't quite right. It was so funny! We also took the kids to see "Megamind", a really funny movie. Daniel would say (REAL LOUD!): "What's happening Mommy??". Thank God there weren't a lot of people there!

Tomorrow we'll decorate gingerbread men cookies and I promise I won't have a quiet internal freak out when the kids get frosting all over the place . . .

The times, they are a changin'

Nov 14, 2010 2:54pm

Lucy's friend slept over last night and even though they stayed up late watching Rapunzel, both girls were awake at 7:30 am. I was in bed trying to convince myself it's morning and I should get up too especially because all the kids are up when I hear Lucy say: "You are my best BFF". MY BEST BFF???? Since when does she know what a BFF is? How did this happen??? She's only 6!!!!! OMG!

What's happening right NOW?

Nov 16, 2010 2:48pm

One of the differences between humans and animals is our ability to anticipate events, to predict what is coming. The problem I have with that unique skill is that I'm not sure it really makes humans superior to other animals. It's true it gives us the ability to plan and prepare . . . but mostly it seems to cause anxiety, ulcers and stress.

My anticipation of surgery, the subsequent pain and inability to play with the kids adequately has been weighing heavily on me. I'm sure it will be manageable, I'm sure the days will pass and I'll soon be able to lead a fairly normal life but the repeating thought has done nothing but crowd my days and create more guilt than I probably need to be feeling.

So today I went back to the lesson I already learned a few months ago: there is a time for everything. Today I'm not having surgery, today I'm enjoying feeling good. When surgery comes on Friday, I'm sure I'll know what to do and when I come back home and the kids want to play, I'm sure I will think of something fun. But right now isn't the time to beat myself up over it. This is my time to be sick with cancer and it's important to accept and embrace it no matter how unpleasant and seemingly unfair it is. Our lives have a certain trajectory regardless of how we feel about it. Fighting that, fighting how our lives are meant to unfold never works . . . nor should it.

Day before surgery

Nov 18, 2010 6:12pm

What a day! We were supposed to have a relaxed day with only 2 short appointments to be done by noon before my surgery tomorrow. We were only done at 3 pm and this after rushing from appointment to appointment so we're both exhausted. From blood tests, to more ultrasounds, to more imaging, we ran from floor to floor trying to get it all done. I decided to participate in 2 more clinical trials so some extra testing and shots also came my way but I keep thinking about Lucy and all her little friends who could grow up and also develop breast cancer. If I can help it be an easier process for them, then I'm happy to!

We report for surgery at 7:30 am where I am given these two shots that are supposed to sting like a bee sting before they get me prepped. My plastic surgeon sees me and decides where he will make incisions and I'll be ready to go. I'll be put to sleep (I hate this part) and for the following 7 to 8 hours the surgeon removes tissue and tests it all for cancer, also removing lymph nodes as needed. After all the cancer has been removed and the main surgeon is confident I'm clear, the plastic surgeon goes to work.

Sigh . . . . wish me luck!

Day before surgery—part II

Nov 18, 2010 9:41pm

I'm back in the hotel after a wonderful dinner out in Rochester. We'll need to get up early so I've wanted to take it easy tonight. I spent the first 10 minutes back here feeling nervous about tomorrow, nervous about being put under and how it'll all feel afterwards. It's probably a better idea to remember the humorous side to all this. My guess is tomorrow will probably have a lot of funny moments . . . I just hope it's not because I say something totally stupid to the surgeons when I'm still groggy! I bet I'll do just that . . . .

Our first meeting with my surgeon today had it's moments. That's when the whole day got off track and a pile of new appointments and tests were placed on my "itinerary". The Mayo calls your list of appointments consisting on needle pricks, sensitive parts of your body getting squished and cut into your "itinerary". Yup . . . . this feels JUST like a tropical vacation! Anyway, this surgeon is awesome and one of the best at the Mayo. But in the same breath as she says "I've done thousands of these things, it'll be just fine" she then says "Who's in charge if something were to go wrong?". I stare at her and slowly point at Steve. What does she mean "if something goes wrong??". What is she implying he's in charge of? The color gown they put on me or something else? (I know, I know, it's just standard procedure).

So after this meeting, where I sign up for the 2 additional clinical trials, I need to provide a blood sample. I've already given enough blood to revive Frankenstein but nonetheless they wanted more. We got there 20 minutes early hoping to get it done quickly but it was so busy that I was late for the appointment I had with the plastic surgeon. Because of my port the nurse accessing it needs to use a fairly large hooked needle that hurts going in. So the lady says "I'll tell you when I'm about to poke, ok honey?". Thank God. I like to be prepared. And then she proceeds to say absolutely nothing and just out of the blue STAB me with the needle. NO warning whatsoever! And the day continued crazily on . . .

Tomorrow I start the day needing to get two injections that sting like bee stings. I had two separate nurses tell me that today . . . just so I'm forewarned. Great. And by the way, the surgeon won't let me stay awake for the surgery. Yes, I asked. She laughed and said I'd be 'bored' if I were awake for the whole 7 hours . . . I think not. I think I could provide keen insight and maybe lighten the mood with some interesting yet funny anecdotes. She still declined.

Surgery

Nov 20, 2010 11:26am

Exactly 24 hours ago they were making their first incision . . . according to Steve, I was totally out of it of course. The surgery was 6 hours but I was only back in my room at 7:45 pm. I long day especially for Steve who had to wait around for updates every 2 hours.

The good news is they found no cancer left in either breast and perhaps some left over in one lymph node but they are waiting for more in depth pathology. All the lymph nodes are gone anyway, so I consider myself cancer free right now and all subsequent treatments are to prevent recurrence. I like my odds!

The plastic surgeon did a phenomenal job . . . . really phenomenal. Frankly I was afraid of seeing myself post surgery and bursting into tears but I still look a lot like I used to.

Now the pain after waking up . . . how do you describe it other than having an elephant sitting on your chest and killer bees stinging your sides. I don't think I've ever been in that much pain but 12 hours later I can walk around and feel MUCH better. They say I look great and could go home today. It's hard to rest here; people keep coming in to take my blood pressure so it wasn't the most restful night. Don't get me wrong, I walk around like a 90 year old lady, feel dizzy a lot and it only hurts when I breathe. Don't read the following if you are squeamish . . . . ready? I have these tubes sewn into me with bulbs at the end to accumulate fluid that needs draining twice a day for 10 to 14 days. It's disgusting!

I really miss the kids but I can't care for them in this state. Thinking of them is what drove me to do this surgery, the clinical trials, all the chemo; and thinking of them is pushing me to do what I need to in order to heal.

Finally home

Nov 20, 2010 9:35pm

We got home around 5 pm and it's nice to be here! There's no resting properly at the hospital with constant interruptions from nurses. They were great but all I really need to do now is manage pain, eat and move around as much as possible. Oh, and nap! I'm exhausted!

Recovery . . .

Nov 21, 2010 8:39pm

I'm starting to return to the world of the living. I'm still extremely sore but have made a point of walking around and staying somewhat busy with frequent breaks so my energy level is still where it needs to be. It's amazing how much surgery takes out of you and the effect the painkillers have. I'm on some pretty strong stuff which I take religiously.

I always knew this surgery was my only option, I couldn't see myself just doing a lumpectomy no matter how hard I tried to convince myself that would be a less radical option. The surgery decision is always very personal and different people feel comfortable with different options; but from the moment I got my diagnosis I knew what I needed to do no matter how much it scared me to go through the actual procedure. The other thing weighing on me was how I'd look afterwards. I told my plastic surgeon I pictured looking like a granade exploded on my chest and was trying to come to terms with that. Well, turns out that's not the case at all. I'm not even done with the reconstruction which takes months and I feel like I not look only human, but female. It's one of those unspoken things women wonder about: will I still look and feel like a woman?

Doctors spend so much time talking about options from a medical perspective that the emotional part can get lost. How will I feel when the nurse first removes the gown to look at the incisions? Will I be brave enough to look down? And when I do, will I still feel and look like me?

The answer is yes, you do.

Cancer gone??

Nov 22, 2010 4:44pm

During surgery the pathologist does a quick test to check for cancer as they proceed with the operation mostly to confirm where the cancer has spread to. In my case we knew all lymph nodes would be taken out because my biopsy pre-chemo was positive; we just didn't know how many were affected.

Where during surgery they felt there was still some cancer left in the lymph nodes removed, the more complete pathology came back today and they didn't find cancer anywhere! Neither breast and none of the lymph nodes.

Looks like the first 12 chemo rounds did their job, even more so than was expected and any further treatments are icing on the cake! Yea!

Lessons

Nov 23, 2010 9:18pm

There are constant lessons as I go through cancer treatment. Obviously it's great to know the cancer is no longer detectable using pathology, it's scary but nice to know I have even more chemo and radiation coming my way to help me feel even more confident that the odds of recurrence are very low but there are never ending challenges no matter what stage in the process a person is in. As you sit in the pre-op room, as you are wheeled into the operating room and there are 20 people there all scrubbing up and glancing at you through their masks, you realize you're truly alone going through it all. It's extraordinarily comforting to read all the messages left on my blog, they often bring tears to my eyes and I can feel the real empathy. All that plays a key role in my ability to keep on going, to keep on fighting this illness. But it's also true for all of us that we are born alone and we will go through many very difficult situations truly alone no matter how many people are on the sidelines cheering us on. When you're lucky someone shows up and gives you a hug letting you know they are there beside you. But ultimately, it's a journey we all make by ourselves.

This has really taught me to pay attention to others and the issues they might be going through that I might blow off or not really notice.

But at the end of the day, get to know and love yourself—you'll spend the rest of your life keeping yourself company.

Giving Thanks

Nov 25, 2010 9:33pm

It's probably not appropriate to just spend one day a year thinking about what all we are thankful for, but I guess today is the chosen day for the entire country to get together and do so . . . hopefully the stereotypical family arguments and the stress over the food all being done at the same time doesn't take away from the meaning of this holiday. I could get all profound and deep, have the traditional list of "thanks" which of course are true for us all. Who would we be without our family? And the kids who make us laugh, keep us up at night worried if they will turn out and melt our hearts? How empty would it feel if we didn't have that special person who puts up with all our little eccentricities? I'm so thankful for all that, for my doctors who rock, my own body who seemed to decide that cancer has no home in here and all the possibilities that lie out there for me after my energy is back.

Then there's little things most of us never think we'll EVER be thankful for . . . . like the fact that I can still frown even though my eyebrows are mostly gone. Very important when your 2 year old decides to dip his fingers in his yogurt.

My wish . . .

Nov 26, 2010 10:47pm

Medically today was a good day. I am in less pain although walking around is still a delicate process and I was able to go down to the Mayo to have 3 of my 5 drains removed. What a huge relief that was! Those drains are heavy, unwieldy to lug around and frankly hurt me. So now I'm only left with two which is more manageable. I'm finally off narcotics too . . . I hate the way those things make me feel although I'd strongly advise anyone going through this to stick to taking them without fail until the pain is under control.

The hardest part having cancer and young children is knowing it's been months of chemo, lots of days when I'm not feeling well, the surgery where I can't really care for them properly, etc . . . and they don't really understand it. I am missing out on playing out in the snow with them (although I did take them once sliding down the hill when the big snow storm came right before surgery). I can't just take them places, pick them up, roll around on the floor and create those precious memories our childhoods are full of. I know healing is my main job right now so that I can be here for them for many years to come but the most painful part of cancer is missing my kids. I can deal with surgery, I can deal with more chemo but I can barely deal with the sense that my children aren't with me and when they are they need to be careful around me. If I had one wish, I'd wish for that back.

The elusive speck . . .

Nov 29, 2010 9:59am

I'm not a very patient person. I'll start off by saying that. Not in the slightest. Ok, so given that immutable fact here goes: I had my surgery on the 19th so I should be way better by now!!!! It's been 10 days already but things still hurt and even though I can reach above my head, I can't stretch my arms fully. Certain positions still hurt and I'm guessing that when I drive today it'll be painful. I can't pick my 2 year old up and would love to take the kids to the movies (which means picking Daniel up so he can sit on the seat), I can't decorate a Christmas tree which I've always loved doing because it's my favorite holiday and I'm just generally feeling extraordinarily irritated that I'm not healing faster! An irritated latin is a really crabby latin!

Ok . . . pity party kinda over . . . .

Here's a nice story though. Last night I was going through my bedtime routine with the kids which ends with the lights off, me on the floor between their beds and each one holds one of my hands. Lucy grabs it with both her hands and snuggles and Daniel wants my hand over his head. We usually talk quietly about whatever is on their mind (mostly mine or Lucy's although Daniel is chiming in now too). Lucy seemed a little sad or worried about me because she knows I hurt a bit right now and she also knows I need to do 4 more chemos. She was adding them up saying I would end up doing 16 "medicine treatments". She knows the cancer is now gone so she asked why I would do 4 more. "To be absolutely sure this never comes back Lucy". "Oh", she said. "Then you should do it just in case there is a little speck of cancer left". So that's my new mantra: I'm doing the extra chemo and 25 radiation sessions, I'm dealing with the surgery pain to get that little speck. Just in case there is that one little speck. It's worth hunting and taking it down!

It's Official

Nov 29, 2010 11:31pm

Tonight I received a letter from the Mayo clinic with the formal results from my surgery, and I quote:

".... you had no evidence of residual viable tumor within the breast and with 24 lymph nodes negative. Overall staging is a ToNo; COMPLETE PATHOLOGICAL RESPONSE".

They had called me earlier and told me they found no cancer after surgery and after removing all the lymph nodes which at one point had tested positive. But to see it written down, in black and white, is such a relief. I don't think I had allowed myself to really believe that at the moment I am cancer free. Obviously all people diagnosed with cancer worry about the tiny speck that might be lurking around and could recur but I am medically cancer free according to the best hospital in the world.

Everything else seems so unimportant when just a few short months ago I feared I could die within a year or two. Now I have evidence of the butt kicking that went on during my chemo! More to come, but it's worth it!

Darn drains . . .

Dec 2, 2010 7:32pm

I'm slowly recovering and the majority of the pain is due to the remaining 2 drains pulling and tugging. I'll definitely need to be on top of my rehab exercises to regain range of motion which is very limited right now . . .

It's amazing how difficult small tasks become after surgery and I don't think I ever really appreciated that, especially people who live with chronic pain or who are for some reason not able to do what the rest of us take for granted.

A simple task like picking Lucy up from school or taking a shower are huge undertakings. I have to really plan ahead and give myself time for things like this now. It took me over an hour to shower today! The first 5 minutes consist of me standing in the bathroom getting up the courage to go through the entire exercise facing me. I need to get something long to use it to push the shower head out . . . something I used to reach up and do in 2 seconds now takes several long painful seconds. And getting undressed takes a lot of planning and forethought. Not falling over is IMPERATIVE (as imperative as not sneezing has been for the past 2 weeks. I absolutely CANNOT sneeze, I can only imagine what that'll feel like and go to great lengths to not need to sneeze). When I finally get into the shower it takes forever! I confess after my 30 minutes trying to soap up, I spend a good 10 minutes standing there under the hot water getting mentally prepared to dry myself. Sometimes I just don't drink for as long as possible because I cant reach my glass! If I forget to ask for a glass before Steve leaves, I'm stuck! And climbing up on a chair is not going to happen! Remember: not falling over . . .

But you also find ways to manage around the difficulties. Like picking up Lucy from school. I kick my car door shut, I keep my seat as far back as I can so reaching the seat belt is even possible. I also confess I always consider skipping it entirely but "if you don't click it, ticket!", right? And what if Steve drives the car before me? And the rear view mirror is not set for me? I've sat in the car for a long time staring at the mirror, willing it to move back enough for me to see out the back but apparently I have no psychic abilities.

I can only get these drains out Monday if all goes well and I'm trying to not let it get me down. 3 more days.

The Drain Saga . . .

Dec 4, 2010 2:11pm

The drains are out! The drains are out! But what an ordeal that was . . . .

I called the Mayo on Thursday telling them one of the two was ready to go and the second would be ready Saturday, but I was willing to drive down Friday to just get one removed! It took the Mayo a long while to get back to me on when on Friday I could get down there for the 3 second procedure of removing the drain but with the winter storm coming I decided to just put up with it until Monday. When I finally spoke with them on Friday they suggested I leave both drains in until Tuesday because I already have a pile of appointments scheduled for Tuesday . . . ARE YOU KIDDING ME? I get that it makes more sense, is waaaay more efficient and what's 4 days in my whole lifetime, but ARE YOU KIDDING ME?

The Mayo had often suggested I have a care giver up here do it. When I had my first 3 drains removed I had tried calling Park Nicollet and after several operators, nurses and conversations with their Breast Center was told they don't that the right people to do this. How is that possible? It's one stitch that needs cutting, then pull. That's extent of removing one of these things! I called Park Nicollet again on Friday after realizing there was no way I could wait until Tuesday with these things hanging from me, doing the cleaning, disinfecting, and not sleeping because they hurt. Again, after talk to a series of different nurses wanting to understand the mystery behind these drains they scheduled me for an appointment today at 10:30 am at a Park Nicollet. I was ecstatic. Completely relieved, only one last night with those horrible things in and liberated from big bulky tubing. Today at 7:56 am I get a phone call from Park Nicollet. They cancelled saying they feel that they don't have the "right person" to do this. That I need to call my OB/GYN to do it. It was the most frustrating, infuriating, mystifying thing ever! Don't mess with a woman who's had drains hanging off her for over two weeks! First of all: how can you cancel on the patient the day of the appointment?! Second: how do you not have the expertise in house to remove a surgical drain used in a myriad of surgeries all over the world?! And third: OB/GYN????? So because this is breast cancer related surgery and breasts are loosely related to the OB world because they are used to nurse babies, THAT is the correct department for me to call?

I ended up calling the hospital and they told me to just go to Urgent Care. Lucy came along to keep me company and we walked into Urgent Care after a 2 minute wait and this young doctor walked in, laughed at how scared all these other people had been of taking my drains out and took a total of 10 seconds to get them both out. THANK YOU RANDOM URGENT CARE DOCTOR! I feel way better and so should Steve. Plan B was to make him do it.

Today . . .

Dec 8, 2010 2:18pm

These past two days have brought me back to some serious introspection following the news of Elizabeth Edwards losing her battle to breast cancer. For those of you in Portugal, she was the wife of a famous politician who was diagnosed with stage III breast cancer around 2004. I think at some point she was considered "cured" but unfortunately it came back in her bones and organs. It had heard two days ago that the doctors decided there was nothing else that could be done and she passed away yesterday at 61.

I don't want to be overly dramatic or let this sad event bring us all down, but I also don't want to ignore it. I have absolutely no doubt that anyone either with cancer, who's been diagnosed with cancer and is in remission or knows someone in that situation was affected by her death. It makes us all stop and realize that it could be any one of us.

There is a time for each and every one of us to leave this earth and I've come to realize it's not always as "far away" an event as we might assume. Coming to terms with that is a long process. No matter how long I have, I think I'll never get enough of my husbands jokes or my kids laughter. Fight for your future as valiantly as you can, but do your very best enjoying today. It's all you really have.

Time to get back to the fight

Dec 8, 2010 10:52pm

When I was in graduate school the Dalai Lama came to the Twin Cities and gave a talk and the U of MN. I was lucky enough to go listen to him and one thing he said stuck with me ever since. He said when we are sad or afraid we try to "get around" those feelings by ignoring them or burying them deep inside. His point was that doesn't work and only leads to other problems. The only way to deal with uncomfortable situations and emotions is to move THROUGH them. So for these past couple of days I've been accepting and genuinely feeling the fear that arose from learning of the death of another breast cancer patient (Edwards). I've felt the fear, I've thought again about all the reasons I think I am still here and all the reasons why I can fight and beat this thing. I've dealt with the event, felt the feelings and am now ready to get back on track. I need to do a better job at eating healthy—I fell off the wagon a little bit these past weeks—and I need to get back to laser focus on healing, staying stress free and enjoying life. I am working hard to regain mobility in my arms so the lack of lymph nodes doesn't become a life long problem and I want to do it before my next chemo treatment starts. A tall order but I think I can do it! And I'm going to take a lot of deep deep breaths during my chemo to make sure it moves through every single cell in my body; hunting down any stray cancer cells that might be plotting to return. I will beat this ugly disease.

I'm no artist . . . .

Dec 10, 2010 7:18pm

Today was the most active I've been since my surgery 3 weeks ago and now I'm exhausted. Driving a manual transmission all morning is probably good exercise for me as I get my arms and chest muscles stronger, but it sure does hurt!

At 2 pm I went to Lucy's gingerbread house building event in her classroom. I went in quite innocently not really imagining this was going to turn into a major construction project. Keep in mind, I'm portuguese and some things we simply don't do back home. Gingerbread houses is one of them. I have never, ever built one and only really know what they are because I've seen them at holiday parties.

The room was filled to the brim with parents and grandparents who gathered around their child's miniature desk. We were given a huge bag filled with candies, pretzels, tiny marshmallows, teddy grahams, smarties, and all sorts of other colorful items. Additionally we all brought a box of Graham Crackers and frosting to build our masterpieces. We let Lucy mostly guide the shape this "house" was going to take. I have the word house in quotes because I look back and think it probably ended up being a gingerbread bunker or warehouse. But Lucy was having a blast, plopping icing on specific key spots she felt needed more "glue" and trying to put a smiley face on its side. This was after the first and only attempt at a roof failed horribly. She ended up with more frosting on her hands, hair, pants, shirt and tummy but overall had a blast. I tried my best but was fairly useless in helping her and it's really meant for the kids to enjoy, spend time with their parents and take home their works of art. We let her do whatever she wanted to while I ate the licorice.

Thankfully we were sitting next to a couple whose house kept collapsing so we all had some laughs. I was feeling as though our "house" was pretty average until I looked around! You should have seen some of these things! Literal mansions with smarties neatly lining the roof, little doors and steps leading up to them, trees in the yard (we had lollipops in our candy bags), even fences. And one of the houses had house numbers above the door. Seriously! House numbers! Perfect tiny miniature cottages! At least we get points for originality thanks to her dad . . . . Lucy had a teddy graham dangling down the side of her "house" tied to a licorice strand. Apparently he'd been putting up Christmas lights and fell off the the roof tangling himself in his string of lights. I bet no one else has a teddy graham facing peril.

Feeling good

Dec 13, 2010 8:16pm

I'm slowly getting my mobility back with the occasional twinge and still tightness in my arms but with time I'm sure I'll be back to normal. Maybe one more week of exercising to stretch this out and I'll be practically done. On Wednesday I have my next oncology and radiation therapy appointments and expect to know a little more about the next steps, more precisely the timing of the chemo. I'm really not looking forward to doing that all over again but will definitely embrace the whole thing. I think if I relax into it, it'll be more effective. I don't know if that's true or not, but it can't hurt, eh?

I'll have to go through my hair falling out again too. It's coming back and I'm so proud of my 3 mm long hair! I still need to wear hats, it's not as though it looks like a "normal" short cut but nevertheless I've enjoyed seeing it. I don't think it's quite the same color though. Initially it looked like it was coming back gray, then oddly enough it changed to dark brown and now . . . . well . . . it's hard to describe. We have a saying in Portugal: it's the color of a donkey running away. A nondescript brownish sort of thing. But hey, I like it! At least it's there! My guess is by end of January it'll be all gone again but by May it'll have returned.

Meanwhile a friend sent me some of her chemo hats and 2 wigs she was going to donate. For those of you following my care pages for a long time you might recall just how much Lucy LOVES wigs. As I type this update I am sitting on my bed watching a Princess Ariel movie with Daniel and Lucy who are cuddled under the covers. Oh wait, did I say Lucy? Forgive me, now it's Princess Jessica who has long flowing dark hair. The second she spotted the wigs she was on it! And don't tell her but she's convinced now Daniel can't recognize her and believes she really IS thing Jessica character.

Emotional Day

Dec 15, 2010 8:40pm

Today was a very emotional day at the Mayo. We had an appointment with radiation oncology to talk about the plan post chemo so a nurse sits down with us and proceeds to go through my history to date. "You found a lump early in the year . . . it appeared negative for cancer but after a 6 month re-check and a biopsy it was determined to be cancer . . .". Why is this lady making me relive this whole thing? "They determined the cancer was invasive, ductal, present in the lymph nodes which meant it spread and triple negative" she continues. At this point I'm really trying to shut her out, it's hard not to go through the emotions I had when all that happened back in July. And then the shocker: "On August 5th you did a PET scan here at the Mayo and they could see the tumor in the breast, under arm lymph nodes and lymph nodes center line chest". WHAT? The cancer was also in the lymph nodes in my chest? No one ever told us that!

At this point terror washes over me and I can't really hear what anyone is saying. Steve is telling them this is news to us and asking why we didn't know, the nurse and a doctor are combing through the PET scan photos showing us the areas highlighted and I'm literally having a silent panic attack. Fortunately Steve had all sorts of questions which I think made it harder for anyone to tell I was losing it. I would nod politely, ask a few questions trying to sound normal but a voice in my head was screaming "If you die in the next year or two your children won't remember you. They won't even remember you".

Panic attack aside, here are the facts. The first PET scan showing cancer traveling to lymph nodes in my chest was done before I started chemo, as a baseline. The second PET scan I did was 15 days into chemo; after only 2 of the 12 chemo cycles I did. That second PET scan shows the tumors in my breast and under arm lymph nodes to be smaller, and the lymph nodes in my chest appear clean already. The radiation oncologist said that my response to chemo was really extraordinary and no one would have expected such a good response. Of course they always remind me that a triple negative breast cancer requires all "tools" at their disposal because they can be harder to treat, etc (panic attack returns when I'm reminded of how dangerous this all is) but results are very encouraging.

Next I go see my oncologist to plan the next round of chemo. That appointment went a LOT better. He said that a complete pathological response is the absolute best one could have hoped for. Essentially we are now only treating recurrence and not trying to "cure" me anymore, that's been done. And although he doesn't like to quote numbers, in a situation like mine recurrence rates are now something like 10%. So I have a 90% shot at never seeing this cancer ever again. 90%! When he first met me, he gently mentioned that triple negatives are traditionally in the 70% range . . . 30% recurrence is the average.

The other "good" news was that where this next chemo drug is notoriously nasty, it's not worse than what I was doing before. He explained the clinical trial regime was especially harsh and that when it becomes standard of care for patients they will 'soften' the treatment giving patients breaks between cycles, lowering the doses, etc. So I know I can handle what they did before; I'll be able to handle this next round particularly if it's only 4 times. I know that when I'm in the throes of it I'll be sick and miserable and feel like it will never end. But I can do this and my kids will remember me.

Starting to put surgery behind me . . .

Dec 20, 2010 4:37pm

I just got back from the Mayo Lymphedema clinic where they checked my left arm for swelling and a physical therapist made sure I'm on track to regain my mobility in both arms. Turns out I'm doing really well and on track to get it all back, which is a good thing. Reaching above my head without feeling like something inside my arms is about to snap loose will be nice . . .

I'll forever need to monitor my left arm however. No lymph nodes means fluid could easily accumulate in it leading to swelling, infection and a long list of horrors. They're on top of it though and this is nothing that can't be managed if it happens. Things are good.

It's nice to start feeling like the surgery chapter is behind me as I walked around the Mayo waiting for my appointment. Not feeling pain all the time is awesome! This really was a much bigger surgery than I expected it was going to be and way more painful than I expected! But it also had it's interesting moments as a friend and I reminisced about our surgeries recently . . .

Before surgery the patients are "prepped" which I thought meant putting them in a gown, starting an IV line and putting them on a bed with wheels to roll them around the hospital from pre-op into the operating room. Nope. As we sit waiting for the IV nurse to come hook me up, a nurse comes in and asks me my name and date of birth. I'm used to this, every nurse at the Mayo will ask you this question no matter what you are there for and before they even do anything else. But then the nurse pulls out a pen, places it on her notebook and asks me: "Can you describe the procedure are you here for?". Huh? Are you asking me what I'm in for? Is this a trick question? If my surgeon lost her notebook, I'm happy to go back home until she finds it!! I'm taken aback and in VERY lay terms explain the procedure "using my own words". Using my own words only really means I have no idea what the medical terms are so I mumble something like "Mastectomy . . . . all lymph nodes are to be taken out on my left side . . . immediate reconstruction with plastic surgery . . . . please sow me back up". Remember that nightmare? You know the one. You are in school taking a test and suddenly realize you forgot to study. What if I don't tell them the correct procedure?! What if I left something out and therefore they don't do it?!

And do you know how many times I was asked this?? There were at least 4 or 5 different nurses asking why I was there and what surgical procedures I'm going to have?! Don't you folks talk to each other? I certainly understand that I need to take charge of my health care but I was under the impression that on the day of surgery I just needed to show up at 7 am and be successfully unconscious for several hours. If they ask me again I'm saying "An oil change and tire rotation".

I do know why they ask and appreciate their efforts making sure that I as the patient am clear on what is going on. I noticed the notepads the nurses and doctors carry around says "The patient comes first" on the bottom. And it shows . . .

Truth and Perception

Dec 21, 2010 12:28pm

It's Daniel's birthday tomorrow—he turns 3! He's moderately excited about it, as best an almost 3 year old can be about something that feels abstract to him. But he does know he'll get a cake and presents, so I suppose he has the gist of it. Meanwhile Lucy had a major melt down, sobbing for a good 20 minutes this morning telling me she doesn't like it when other people get presents and she doesn't. I was truly amazed that she literally said "First I feel jealous, then I feel mad and then I don't like the person ever ever ever ever again!" . . . and she'd bawl some more. Watching such a little kid be so aware of what she's feeling, be able to articulate her feelings and accept them is truly a talent that will serve her well through her life. I was so proud of her. I'm 37 and still trying to pinpoint what I'm feeling half the time! I remember being a kid and watching other kids getting stuff I wasn't getting and how that felt. How do you explain to a little kid that she needs to be happy for other people sometimes too? How do you explain that this obsession with 'stuff' isn't the key to being happy anyway? And this from the woman who is probably the largest contributor of all the toys we have lying around here?! I'd buy toys for all 4 kids everyday if I could . . . Our perception is that buying things makes us happy but the truth is it doesn't. Buying something can be fun, don't get me wrong. I enjoy it too. A lot. But I'll always remember when last weekend we all sat by the fireplace after having brownies and watched a funny movie together. That's the real deal!

Meanwhile, I've been trying to reconcile the truth versus my perceptions about my cancer from day one. You're sitting in your office, worried about your next meeting, wondering what you'll make for dinner, certain that you'll be around when your kids are adults (not that you ever think about it, it's a given) and you're feeling healthy. Then your phone rings and a voice you don't know tells you they found cancer and you need to come see the surgeon tomorrow. So you stand up, walk out and drive home. And all of a sudden everything changes because someone told you it did. Not because you feel different or sick, but because of one phone call from a stranger. Actually accepting I was one of the people who has cancer has been a process. I fluctuated between moments of pure terror (my perception) and moments of acceptance (the truth).

And now people I've met only a few times in my life tell me it's gone. The cancer isn't there anymore they said. It's great news, wonderful news and taking me a while to accept and relax into news. I don't feel any different now either. I just got used to the notion that this ugly thing is inside me and now they say it's not there . . . . so I find myself repeating "It's gone. It's really gone. It's gone. It's really gone. You're going to be ok". Feels a bit like whiplash.

Getting tons of toys will make us happy and that feels like the truth. It's not. Living the rest of your life afraid of recurring cancer can also feel like the truth. It's not.

The best season . . .

Dec 26, 2010 7:32pm

This past week was great! Christmas is my favorite time of the year, hands down. I love the Christmas lights, love the corny Christmas music and I even eat fruit cake. I'm one of those people who have 99% of my shopping done by the first week in December and all presents wrapped several days before Christmas eve. That's probably the most painful task if you ask me . . . wrapping . . . I hate wrapping. For the first hour I'm still chirpy as I imagine the recipient of the said gift opening it and exclaiming "It's just what I wanted!", or "Eeeeeeeeeeeekk! An easy bake oven!!!!!!!!!". But by the third hour of cutting and folding and taping festive paper over increasingly more challenging gifts my brain starts to play tricks on me: "C'mon Joana, no need to be perfect . . . in fact, no one will notice if you just shove it in a Target bag and tape that shut". Into the fifth hour of wrapping I'm in a boredom induced coma.

But now it's all done, the gifts are open, the kids behaved wonderfully and seemed to really love their gifts. Yes, I love Christmas!

And tomorrow I'll be thrown back into the reality of my treatment not being done yet. At 8 am we drive back down to Rochester for my first chemo treatment in 2 months. To be honest I've been planning this upcoming week as if the chemo treatment will barely affect me—a big mistake, I get it. It's the oddest thing but when you're well you really have a hard time picturing being sick . . . and similarly when you are sick you have a hard time remembering healthy. It's really wasn't all that long ago that just drinking water made me nauseous and walking upstairs was a huge effort. But now here I am thinking about taking the kids bowling and to the Science Museum next week. My master plan is to continue to ignore the fact that chemotherapy is the most toxic type of treatment out there and deal with it as it comes. The silver lining is that instead of weekly, this time my treatments are every two weeks. More days feeling good! Yippee!

Hopefully you all had a wonderful and peaceful Christmas. It's the perfect time to remember the things we should be appreciating every single day of the year. I've come to discover life is fragile and our real strength comes in the depth of the relationships we have. Such a blessing . . . . who's the blessing in your life?

Chemo horrors . . .

Dec 28, 2010 5:11pm

We went down to the Mayo yesterday to complete the genetics testing that will tell us definitively whether or not I have the "breast and ovarian cancer" gene followed by the first chemo treatment. I had to hold back tears most of the day because now I know what's coming and chemotherapy drugs are nasty! As I sat there listening to the IV pump going, pushing these noxious drugs inside me I had a flash that I really sort of get to choose how happy or unhappy I am going to be regardless of my situation. I'm not always able to fully control that yet, but I get glimpses into the truth that is: we can decide to feel joy no matter what is going on outside of us. And I held on to that for a long while until we got back to the Twin Cities and suddenly I feel a wave of darkness go over me. The funny thing with chemo drugs is they literally do something to your brain. A friend of mine refers to it as entering the Valley of Darkness. It's so true. Shortly after I felt a little bit of pain all over my body along with a sensation of fragility. If someone bumps into me I'll disintegrate. And the last, most unpleasant feeling of all: the most powerful nausea I've ever experienced, and I'm one of those women who get so sick when I'm pregnant that I need IV fluids. This was way worse. We barely made it home in time for me to rush to the bathroom and I was sick every 60 seconds or so from 5 pm until 8 pm. All the nausea drugs in world weren't helping me at all—and believe me the Mayo gave me a huge arsenal of drugs to help fight it off. It got so bad I had to take a blanket into the bathroom and doze in there between waves of being sick. It's this surreal state when you are so tired you can hardly stay awake so when you close your eyes you start dreaming these odd goofy dreams, only to be yanked back into the real world with a new wave of nausea. At 8:15 Steve crushed one of the nausea pills so I could at least have some hope of it going into my blood stream and working. I think I was getting past the worst of and was able to get that medicine inside me. I went straight to bed and slept most of the night.

I had to go back to the Mayo today just for my Neulasta shot—it helps my body make white blood cells that get killed during chemo. It's a long drive when you are still feeling very sick and fairly weak but I have no choice but to go. It's this shot that allows them to give me chemo every other week instead of every 3 weeks. The nurses back at the chemo unit were very kind today. A few came to seek me out as I waited for this shot to be ready, having heard I'd had a rough night. I guess most people don't react quite as strongly but they might have a few tricks up their sleeves for my next treatment. I really need next time to be easier that this—it's truly awful. I have no energy, which I expected. Feel like I've been hit by a truck, which I expected. My brain plays tricks on me by telling me I'll never feel ok EVER again, which I also expected. But the strength of the nausea and not keeping anything down was a surprise. My first chemo rounds knocked me on my rear . . . . this round knocked me on my back.

Coming out of it . . .

Dec 29, 2010 1:38pm

I think I'm feeling a little bit better today—finally! It's still a bit touch and go, certain smells set me off and I rush to the bathroom but overall it's under control. I think one of the hardest things, as usual, is my inability to be the "normal" mom I used to be. When you have no energy, feel this sick and everything hurts, you just know you're not fun or doing a good job as a parent. Mid Feb seems like such a long

long way away right now . . . my kids deserve better than this and it's so unfair that cancer affects the whole family like this.

A new day tomorrow

Dec 29, 2010 10:49pm

Ok—that's it. I'm tired of being sick and I think I'm fighting off the side effects now. Tomorrow I'm taking the kids to the IMAX theatre to see a cool movie about life in the ocean and after I might take them to a photo booth to get our photos taken. I love those $3 photo strips you can get at the mall, half fuzzy, half faces, goofy smiles. I've done it ever since Lucy was very little and now Daniel, Lucy and I have occasionally taken them. I need to be creating more smiles around here . . . .

Remembering why

Jan 3, 2011 3:26pm

There are numerous studies on Happiness most of which show that humans aren't very competent at predicting what is going to make them happy which is why we often think it's things like more money, the next thing that strikes our fancy, that next promotion . . . and invariably we're wrong. Imagine two groups of people who are offered a painting from a large selection of beautiful prints. Half the people are told their choice is final and the other half are told they can change their mind and exchange their prints within a week. The study shows that the people who cannot exchange their paintings are significantly happier with their choice than those who can return theirs. Isn't that interesting? If you have no other choice, you are able to accept and feel real happiness with what you have.

I think of those people with real physical disabilities who thrive regardless and are usually full of joy anyway.

Happiness is very simple. It's inside ourselves, it's accepting where you are right now and knowing that's just fine, it's being grateful and being kind to others, it's letting go of anger and struggles for control and then it's about keeping that up. It took me having no choice but to fight for my life to realize this, which is largely why I think I was given my cancer. Here's to not having choices!

Almost done . . .

Jan 9, 2011 7:43pm

Tomorrow I'm off for another full day at the Mayo. It's amazing what they fit into a day! Plastic surgery, rehabilitation, oncology consultation and then 3 hours of chemo. I'm pretty nervous about it and really hoping we can figure out how to make this time less miserable. I guess if it's the same, I'll still make it through though.

I can feel my head itch slightly, an early sign my hair is getting ready to leave me again. *Sigh* . . . . I was getting used to not feeling quite as cold on my head. Oh well.

I realize it's a little short sighted to focus my attention and concern on how I'm going to be feeling tomorrow and early next week. I've also been looking ahead and preparing myself for life after treatment. It often takes me a while to figure out what's going to be an issue and how I might deal with those issues. I started dealing with the emotion of the surgery and reconstruction a couple of months before I was actually going to have it happen and now I'm starting to deal with what might be the future challenges once I'm patted on the back and sent home after my last radiation session sometime late March/early April. If you know anyone who had cancer and is now "cured" understand that for them the ordeal hasn't ended. Everyone has moved on, everyone else breathed a sigh of relief and went back to normal. But for the patient there is no normal anymore. The sense that mortality is very close and never goes away, the knowledge that cancers return in a more deadly fashion is ever present and trying to live a normal daily life as the new person you become through this treatment requires some adjustment. I have definitely changed!

As I look to the future and the happily-ever-after challenge of suddenly being "abandoned" by the army of doctors it's becoming clear that if I feel as though I'm in some sort of control, it'll be easier. I've taken a long hard look at my diet and decided to make some serious changes. I think this is pretty common among cancer patients. We can control what we eat, so there's an area where I can do some real good for myself and feel as though I am still fighting recurrence. I fantasize about swimming in a pool of melted chocolate while eating a slice of chocolate cake topped with whipped cream It's going to be a rough few weeks as I wean myself off my love of desserts, but sugar feeds cancer cells.

It's been really nice to have been able to stay home this whole time and I'm really enjoying and savoring these next few months before I return to work. I'm taking Daniel to a weekly Mommy and me music class (the kid LOVES music) and I've had so much fun being able to take Lucy to school, walk in with her, help her get her stuff together, she loves showing me her desk and all the people she knows. Not rushing out the door in the morning is nice too! I get to usher everyone out and then sit peacefully and drink my tea or coffee . . . of course, those are the days I'm not throwing up, feeling poisoned or unable to get off the couch because of fatigue! Hahaha . . .

I think I'm able to just enjoy this "stay at home mom" thing because I know it will come to an end (just like life: we enjoy it way more if we actually understand and believe it will come to an end . . . we don't always really get that). And to be honest, I'm starting to also get excited about returning to work. It will be interesting to see how all this changes me there but as I look to it now I get the real sense that I'll still be as pumped up about the things that I really care about but with way less stress and better perspective. I think I had a pretty healthy work-life balance before all this but I did become overly stressed and worked up over certain things. Those emotions really don't help you do a better job, in fact they just get in the way. So good riddance! I'll definitely be more present with people too. That's a long lost art nowadays . . .

Hoping for the best . . .

Jan 10, 2011 4:53pm

Here I am in the chemo unit waiting for the IV nausea drugs, steroids and chemo meds to arrive and get the infusion started. It's interesting they call it an "infusion" . . . . you literally feel as though you are sopping wet in this stuff by the end. This is going to sound gross, but if you cough, you can taste it in your mouth as if your cells are oozing this nasty stuff. Ick.

I'm trying hard to not talk myself into feeling nauseous but I can tell I'm playing mental games with myself. Just what I need! Nasty drugs AND my own brain conspiring to make me sick. Good grief . . .

Back home . . . .

Jan 10, 2011 9:50pm

Ok . . . . we made it home. I made us a HUGE salad for dinner followed by my home made soup. All loaded up with healthy fresh vegetables and a few slices of chourizo (a portuguese smoked sausage) for flavor. I'm still considering making myself a smoothie later on: banana, blueberries and yogurt. I'm cautiously optimistic and trying to pretend that last time I felt good and then it hit me out of the blue. Nevertheless I think this is progress right here. Dare I provoke the Gods by declaring this seems to be working better than last time . . . .

One night down . . . .

Jan 11, 2011 12:56pm

After dinner last night Steve and I watched some TV and went to bed. I was feeling pretty ok, just tired and as far as I can tell went right to sleep! I woke at 3 am, thank you steroids!, and sat wondering if I was also getting nauseous. After 3 minutes sitting there . . . yup . . . I was getting nauseous. So Steve was nice enough to get out of bed, go downstairs and bring me my selection of pills to decide the lucky winner. I took one and went back to sleep!

When I woke up this morning I was still feeling very tried (I had hoped to go to the gym today, but that'd be crazy, I don't think I could walk for more than 5 minutes today). I took another pill and made a healthy smoothie and toasted english muffin for breakfast.

Today I need to return to the Mayo just to get a silly sub subcutaneous shot that I could give myself in 3 seconds. But nope! If the pharmacy turns it over to ME, and not a trained nurse or something, then I get charged $6000 administration fee. $6000 to jab yourself, press the tip and be done! At least the drive down will be fun!!

Busy day . . .

Jan 12, 2011 9:04am

I've signed up for a busy day today. In about 20 minutes I'm taking my step son Sam out for breakfast so we can hang out a bit before school. After that I need to go to Daniel's doctors to drop off paperwork to enroll him in a new preschool. After that I'm hitting the gym for a little weight training to get my arm strength back after surgery and try to gently walk on the treadmill . . . . by then I might be too tired but I'm going to give it a shot. Finally I am hoping to go buy some more fresh veggies before returning home and crashing on the couch :o)

Feelin' good!

Oh the indignity . . . .

Jan 13, 2011 1:29pm

I was in the shower today getting ready to take Lucy to school and then Daniel to a toddler music class for his first time, and that's when that dreaded moment arrived. My hair started to come out in huge clumps. I'm never going to get used to that . . . it just would not let up. I've had a lot of pain on my head and neck, usually a sign. But when it finally starts to happen it's just a tiny bit cruel. Hair's just hair, I know. But darn it, I was getting fond of my eyebrows, not looking like a chemo patient anymore. I might have to shave it off instead of watch it fall off in droves and get all over my carpet and couch.

Well, at least it was fun to take Daniel to his music class. He's so proud he goes to music class! He even hugged at kissed me throughout the class . . . so cute.

When it was over he was so disappointed! "WHY WE HAVE GO NOW??? I want to drum some more . . . I want to sing more!". We had to listen to the class CD the whole way home and even once back he had to re enact the little dance sequences he had just learned.

More music

Jan 13, 2011 5:51pm

Today's been a bit rougher, but no big deal. The nausea pills cause headaches which are a little annoying but other than that it's been a good day. At 2:30 Steve, Daniel and I went to the kids school to watch the 5th grade concert. Anthony plays saxophone and all the other grades (Lucy and Sam) we there to watch it too so we got to hang out.

Those 5th graders were playing these instruments for the first time this year but did an amazing job playing together and staying in tune. I was really impressed . . .

They played all sorts of songs, the most memorable being a fancy version of Old MacDonald. The song ended and my 3 year olds voice could be heard sailing across the gymnasium; singing at the top of his lungs "EEEE-IIIIII-EEEEE-IIIIII-OOOOOOOOOOOOOOOOOOOOOOOOOOO!".

Lots of laughs from teachers . . . . they only encourage him . . . .

Bad hair day

Jan 15, 2011 8:24pm

Today was one of those days that I'll look back on and laugh. I'm not sure when exactly I'll be laughing, but I trust I will.

I woke up with little half inch hairs in my mouth which is extremely irritating. My hair insists on flying off and getting inhaled, and I expect to cough up a hair ball any minute now.

I took my morning shower hoping I could just wash it all off and be done, but despite the handfuls of hair I still wasn't anywhere close to bald. But here's the kicker, it doesn't exactly fall out evenly either. Ever seen those National Geographic documentaries about penguins? You know those fluffy cute baby penguins? So adorable and fuzzy. There's a point in the baby penguins life when that fuzz starts to fall off and adult feathers come in. Big bits of fluffy feathers molting off in totally random fashion . . . . yeah, I looked like that. Some parts of my head were full and some getting balder. Nice, eh?

So half way through the afternoon I decided to take another shower but no progress. Lots of hair fell out but I still looked just as stupid. Eventually Steve convinced me to bite the bullet and just shave it off. Off I went for shower number 3 of the day. I was ready with shaving cream and a razor, took a deep breath and proceeded to jam the razor in my hair where it got stuck. Great. I've done this before, I should know by now that first you need the clippers, THEN you shave it. So out I get, dry off and Steve uses the clippers to get my hair down to just a few millimeters long. Of course this exercise has me covered in tiny hairs all over again (along with the bathroom floor). As much as it pains me to admit it, but I need another shower! First to wash off the hairs from pretty much ALL over me, and second to shave my head properly. At this point I'm tired and feeling really dizzy after a long day and 3 hot showers, so my patience was thinning. I shaved the front and top of my head and frankly got too tired to really do the back all that well. Who cares, it's going to be gone in a day or two anyway. It's been a long day! I woke up looking like a teenage penguin and will go to bed looking like a white supremacist without a mirror.

The flood gates opened . . .

Jan 18, 2011 5:25pm

I didn't believe kids actually had temper tantrums in public. I'd read about it but didn't believe it actually happened. Lucy never really went through the terrible twos and threes (fours was a bit of a different issue) and Daniel, although a little more prone to throwing himself on the floor for a few seconds at home, never EVER did it in public. But today, at the doctors office, Daniel had the most furious meltdown.

He was tired so I carried him in from the parking lot and he didn't want to be put down so I pretty much pulled out his insurance card and paid while still holding onto to him. If the payment gets rejected it's most likely because my signature on the receipt looks totally fake and shaky!

The diaper hit the fan when he had to take his jacket, hat and shoes off to be weighed and measured. I was literally wrestling with a little kid who threw himself on the floor crying and shouting that his jacket was NOT coming off. And he's a strong little guy! When he curls up into the fetal position, screaming up a storm, bright red, kicking his legs and tucking his chin under there is no way that jacket is coming off. No way. So I tried to reason with him and explain he needed to help me out. Nope. So I calmly told him he would not be able to watch his movie after we got home like I had promised. "I don't wanna watch movie" he just said. I tried to bribe him telling him about the sticker and candy after the visit. He just shook his head while sucking on his hand and still grasping his jacket like his life depended on it. So I did want any mother ends up doing. I put his Thomas toy in my purse, pulled his shoes off and shoved those in my purse, took his hat off and shoved that in my purse too. I grabbed my overflowing purse, my huge winter jacket and the doctors questionnaire in one hand and literally picked my son up with my other hand tucking him under my arm and carried him like a sac of potatoes over to the baby scale where he could just be plopped on. Holy Smokes! I got my exercise for the day, I can tell ya that. This whole incident lasted for about 5 minutes and afterwards he was his usual cooperative self with the doctor. Interestingly enough he remembered the bribes and promptly asked for his stickers and demanded TWO candies after we were done. This is all my fault of course. The poor little guy was clearly tired and I probably should have rescheduled. He was actually kinda cute as he lay there not being talked into surrendering his jacket.

I did try to ignore the looks of pity. Initially I thought the nurses felt bad for me that I was dealing with this but it honestly doesn't really bother me. But then one of them made a comment about whether or not I felt up to dealing with this given that . . . you know . . . . as she pointed at my head. Clearly the chemo patient, I guess. I'm actually perfectly fine and need to remember that for other people it probably isn't as "normal" as it's become for me. I was also reassured numerous times that the shots Daniel was getting were ok for "people like me". It's always a bit of a shock to see myself through other people's eyes. But I feel good. I swear!

Chemo Cycle #3

Jan 24, 2011 4:58pm

After today's chemo round I'll be left with one last one—hooray! I'm trying not to be too nervous about the nausea this time around. I have one awful and one fairly easy cycle under my belt. I'd like to think that the odds are in my favor this time too since they increased the steroids. The mental part is a challenge though. It's amazing how powerful that is! Just driving to Rochester was hard. The closer to the Mayo I got, the more nausea I felt. It's pretty common for patients to have this, so much so that they give you specific nausea meds for "anticipatory nausea", as they call it.

My visit with my oncologist went well too . . . your typical check-in appointment. He started to question the need for radiation in my situation. My surgeon had also expressed some surprise that radiation oncology was still recommending radiation for me. The more we talk to people the clearer it becomes that the doctors aren't quite sure what to do with situations like mine. My oncologist said that we know radiation is effective in people with more than 3 lymph nodes involved (I only had one), had a lumpectomy (I had a mastectomy) and had the tumor removed via surgery (I had a complete pathological response). There is apparently very little data on people who respond fully to chemo so it's hard to predict the benefits of radiation for someone like me. Of course, the my radiation oncologist has mentioned she'd feel more comfortable with my having the 25 sessions given the type of breast cancer I have. There are 2 things we know work on my type of cancer, and two things alone: chemo and radiation. So let's just do it all because one never really knows if someone is cured from cancer. You only know someone was cured when they die of something else. We need to consider the side effects of the treatment but for the most part I'm prepared to do it all. My only slight concern is the effect on my heart but I'm scheduled to see a cardiologist because of a couple of symptoms I'm experiencing and because my heart has always had goofy rhythm to it. But then again, I always knew I was goofy.

My plan for today: eat nuts and dried fruits as they give me the chemo. I don't want that saline taste in my mouth, always a precursor to the nausea. Let's see if this helps too. A gal has to try SOMETHING to get control over situations like these.

Not shouting "Europe" over the toilet

Jan 25, 2011 9:57am

By the time we got home I could already feel the drugs making me a lot weaker and fragile. I start to walk around like I'm 80 years old but that's been pretty much it. I've not had to throw up which is a huge blessing! I slept really well, woke up still feeling very old but ate a good breakfast. I hope the steroids I took this morning will help me and I'm carrying my nausea pills with me at all times.

At 11 I'm going to an acupuncture appointment and then in the afternoon that long trek back to the Mayo for my 30 second Nulasta shot. I'm a teeny tiny bit tired of driving down there . . . .

The best yesterday was Daniel calling me on the phone because he missed me and Lucy wanting to say hi. She did confess to me once that she likes to talk to me on chemo days to "see if I'm ok". I know she worries a lot about that, but tries to play it cool with me.

All I really have

Jan 26, 2011 1:09pm

I was back at the Mayo yesterday getting my Nulasta shot. The shot that helps me boost my white blood cells after chemo knocks them all out. The nurse who gave it to me happened to be the one who started me on my very first chemo back in August. The unit isn't very big so you end up chatting with them all throughout your treatments and they get to know you. As I was leaving, she turned to grab my arm and said: "You know Joana, you've done really well through all this. Really well.".

These little pats on the back mean so much! For whatever reason, it really matters to me to feel as though I've done well. I had to give some thought to what "done well" means for me and I think I've done well too. It doesn't mean never having been scared, it's important to acknowledge and feel the fear of having cancer. Shoving my head in the sand would not have felt brave. It doesn't mean always doing or saying the right thing to those close to me, I've certainly had my moments of being crabby. But in the long run how has this all transpired? I've grown a lot, I faced things I spent my entire life being afraid of, I come to appreciate the blessings in my life in a way I had never been able to prior and I became closer to my family and friends. I've wondered why it matters to me so much. Why does it matter to me so much the way in which I go through difficult situations. Ever since I was a little kid I believed that when you die you are provided a moment of clarity where you're shown who you really were in life. Not who you tried to be or who you tried to convince others and yourself you were. But the person you actually were. The person we have such a hard time being objective about as humans.

So to some extent I always hope I can go through life with grace and dignity. For years those are the two words that come to mind in any difficult situation. Grace and dignity. If we don't have how we conduct ourselves through life, what else do we really have?

Preparing for the last chapter

Jan 28, 2011 11:44am

I've been reading up on radiation so I can see what I'm getting myself into next. It's nice to know my oncologist is wondering if I really need to do it; I take that as a sign of confidence in my recovery but I'm taking the radiation oncologist's advice and doing it anyway. Radiation appears to decrease recurrence rates and with my age and type of cancer, it's best to just go all out. The side effects are a little scary of course. The radiation needs to hit my chest wall and lymph nodes but not touch my heart. Not touch my lungs. Not touch my spinal cord. Not touch my brain. Hmm . . . .

They make this thing for me to sit in which sets to a given position so that for each of the 25 sessions I'll have the same posture. It takes about a week of mathematical iterations for the oncologist to program this huge sci-fi like machine to shoot and bend rays across my body, hitting the key areas and more importantly, NOT hitting other key areas. Other than some skin burning I don't expect many side effects. After it's all been programmed I get to sit in my special spot, trying not to move at all, praying to the Gods of Trigonometry and hoping this huge thing spinning around me is doing its job . . . I'm sure I'll do what thousands of people have done before me. I'll look through the thick glass separating me from the radiation technician and say: "Beam me up Scottie".

Attack of the killer germs

Feb 1, 2011 11:29am

I finally succumbed to a virus. I've had a stuffy nose for weeks but it had't really affected me much so I thought I'd make it through chemotherapy without actually getting sick. I was wrong. When you don't have an immune system, a run of the mill cold can REALLY suck. Ugh. I can feel my body trying to fight it but not doing a wonderful job! Under normal circumstances this would just be a minor irritation but today my head hurts, I can't stop coughing and I can't breathe.

This has made Lucy be extra attentive with me, rubbing my back and getting me pillows as I was getting her ready in the morning. She does such a good job taking care of me but I do wonder if she worries a little too much about me. I tell her often that I'm just fine and chemo isn't so bad. But I can tell she worries even though she keeps a happy demeanor. How do I balance telling her I'm proud of her for being so helpful but at the same time playing down these symptoms. It's not her job to take care of me, it's my job to take care of her and it's important for kids to have a mother they can count on to protect them no matter what.

It still saddens me to see the kids have to deal with this. Sam walked in the house the other day and the first thing he told me was how he was telling a teacher at his school that I have breast cancer. "She was very interested to hear about it" he said. I think he knows I'm going to be ok, but I wonder what kids are really thinking.

Lucy had an event at her school, a charity event for kids with cancer. In her class they watched a video about kids with cancer and I think they only shared positive stories. Apparently she told some kids (I'm sure for the 100th time :o) that I have cancer and this one kid asked her if I had survived. It' funny because this kid sees me a lot. So Lucy tells me "I told Nick that you had survived and he said he was SO happy because that means you're a survivor!! . . . . Mom . . . . what's a survivor?". Hahaha. I then spend 10 minutes trying to remind her that the cancer is gone. She still talks about it as if I have cancer and I know it's because I'm still doing treatments. In her mind the cancer will be gone when the treatments are done. April. She knows April.

My cancer is bigger than me

Feb 4, 2011 11:26pm

I'm still a little surprised by something that happened this evening. Lucy is in girl scouts, she's a Daisy. And to kick off Girl Scout Cookie selling season there's a big Cookie Dance with all troops. It's really fun, very loud, zillions of little girls all dancing in a church basement. It's the cutest thing! Lots of Taylor Swift and Justin Bieber, lots of disco lighting and probably lots of damage to my hearing.

A few older girls in their early teens are dressed up as cookies and mingle with the girls who are all probably between 6 and 9 years old. The rest of the people are the moms who stand around trying to chat through the noise and some of us occasionally go dance with our kids for a bit. It's hard not to go dance for a bit, belting out the latest Black Eyed Peas hit.

Towards the end of the event one of the older girls, dressed as a thin mint, came over and touched my arm. I honestly thought she had mistaken me for someone because she pulled me aside and said she wanted to thank me for coming.

"Me? You're thanking me?" I was confused. I was standing with two friends, also moms of girls but somehow this young lady is thanking ME for coming. I really thought she was confusing me with someone else.

"Yes. I wanted to thank you for taking the time to come and be here for these girls"

"Me?? Why?"

She sort of teared up and had a hard time talking all of a sudden.

"I'm not sure why you are thanking me. Of course I came, my daughter is a Daisy"

So she said "I don't mean to be offensive, but don't you have cancer?"

"Yes, I have breast cancer. Are you thanking me for coming because I have cancer?"

This is when she really became emotional and started crying. She told me her grandmother had died of cancer and how close they were. That it meant a lot to her to see people with cancer still being there for children. I confess I was still a bit taken aback and kept telling her that of course I was there. That cancer really clarifies what's important, who is important. I hugged her and told her it meant a lot to me that she took the time to come tell me this. I ended up thanking her as much as she was thanking me.

I was stunned as I returned to my two friends. One of them said something along the lines of "it's amazing what you end up representing for other people now". All I could think was "I'm just 'Lucy's mom'". But what this friend said to me stuck with me the rest of the evening . . . she's actually a very wise woman and I tend to listen when she says something. I think she's right. Now I get to represent something to people. I'm under no illusion that it's about me personally because I am truly just Joana, doing what any other person would do in my place. I went to my daughters cookie dance, I take my son to music class, I take all the kids to all sorts of places and love it. I might feel faint at times, I might throw up before I leave the house and frankly not even mention it to anyone anymore because it's no big deal. Lots of people deal with worse, a lot worse. But I can understand the notion of representing something for people.

When I was returning to the Mayo for probably the third time, way back in the beginning of August when I was still in a daze over my diagnosis and trying to keep my head above water I had a 2 minute encounter I still think about today. When you have breast cancer they give you a special binder to keep all information in, so I used to carry mine around those first few appointments. When we walked into the elevator going from the parking ramp into the Mayo clinic there was a woman already in there. She looked at my binder, gave me a big smile and said "I have one of those. Today I'm coming in for my one year check-up. You'll be fine." And I believed her. She had gotten through this thing I was about to embark on, and she told me I was going to be fine. She HAS to be right. She was so certain about it. I've remembered that moment often and assigned that woman some sort of mystical knowledge. To me she represented more than hope, she represented a certainty that I'd be fine.

So how do I deal with my representing something more for some people? I know I wish I had talked to that girl for a bit longer. I could have done a better job consoling her about her grandmother and next time this happens I will do that. See I don't want to belong to some special club of survivors who look inward and pat ourselves on the back over our survivor-ness. But if it means being something positive for those who are just starting down the long road of cancer treatment, or for those who have lost a loved one to cancer or even for those who have to stand by and watch a loved one fight cancer; well, I can do that. There's a role I'm happy to take on. I know I'm just Joana, but if I can gracefully remind a young girl of how much her grandmother loved her it's something worth honoring as best I can.

My final chemo

Feb 7, 2011 1:04pm

I guess I'm graduating. That's how the chemo unit nurse put it when she realized today is my last chemo. They gave me a couple of gift cards and a really nice pin with the words "Celebrate Life" on it.

Driving down here I had moments of real happiness at the thought of doing my last chemotherapy although the side effects don't usually subside until about a week has gone by. But for the most part I'm just a mess of emotions. I think I've had tears in my eyes from the minute I woke up. Not sad tears, just tears.

We met with my oncologist for the last time first thing in the morning. I won't need to see him again until I come in for regular check-ups so it was sort of a good-bye. He told me that recurrence with a lot of cancers can happen anywhere from a year to 10 or even 15 years out but my type of breast cancer will typically either recur within the next 5 to 7 years, or not at all. He also told me I get to feel all sorts of twinges, pains and aches like any other person, so in other words, try not to freak out over every little thing.

I'm not exactly sure how to thank these doctors and nurses. I need to give this some thought later on. Right now I'm trying really hard not to burst into tears every time someone so much as smiles at me. The last chemo, the 16th chemo, is turning out to be a lot more emotional than I had expected.

Final chemo—part II

Feb 7, 2011 8:13pm

It was pretty much a non stop stream of tears during my drive back. I know I still have radiation ahead of me but I sense that won't really be much of a challenge. It'll be an activity I come do but I'm not sure I'll have as much emotion associated with it. It's there to give me some considerable percentage points in the way of survival so definitely worth it's while.

My tears came from looking back at all this. My relief over the complete response, my gratitude over the talent of the plastic surgeon, how touched I was with the bedside manner of my oncologist and my surgeon. Both looking me in the eye, allowing me to cry early on and waiting for me to have "a moment". All those chemo unit nurses who know my name, wave at me as they walk by, always have a laugh to share and always tell me I'm doing well. But I wasn't only crying over the medical aspects of the cancer. I cried over what this has done to the people close to me. I know I scared my husband more than he ever wanted to be scared. I can barely imagine the stress of standing idly by, having your own doubts and fear only to watch your wife express those exact fears. Did he wonder if he'd have to watch me take my last breathes? We never spoke in those terms, but I can imagine what might have gone through his mind in the early months. I'm sure it was hard for him to have to be the caregiver when he too was feeling under attack by the disease. It's ended up making us better and stronger together. Plenty of couples are destroyed by breast cancer . . . I'd give anything to have kept this from my husband but there is part of me that actually sees us closer because of this. That's a good thing. We gained a deeper understanding of ourselves and he helped me in very real ways get through this. Day in and day out. The "I love you and I'm proud of you" as we walk into the elevator after chemo means the world to me. I'm lucky.

I cried because of the people close to me who were scared for me. I can't begin to count the number of people who cried with me, feeling just as vulnerable as I was. I'm sorry I put you through that. I cried because I think in some way this was a bit hard for my kids dad who always offered to help us out in any way we needed and reassured me Lucy and Daniel were handling things just fine from his perspective when he had them. That was always a relief to know and a relief to know I could count on him if I needed it. I'm sad I put him through this too as cancer is an illness that touched his life in a personal and devastating way not long ago. I'm guessing this was the last thing he wanted to have to deal with.

My tears were also for all the people reading my blogs, standing right next to me as I go through this. Whether you write to me or not, I do see you there. And knowing you are there has made all the difference . . . . knowing that you are there regardless of whether you felt comfortable posting anything.

The stress I put my Mom through has also saddened me. She has put on a brave face and been my biggest cheerleader this whole time but I can hardly imagine how it really feels to watch your daughter go through breast cancer when you live across the ocean. If I think of Lucy going through this, it's almost more than I can take.

I cried for my kids who actually seem to be dealing with it all so well. I'm so proud of them! Anthony and Sam are older and smart enough to grasp some of the realities of cancer. But they talked about it in the beginning with me and came to the conclusion that everything was going to be fine. They've adapted wonderfully and didn't distance themselves from me one little bit—something I'd have found normal. Lucy and Daniel remained their usual selves too. In the case of the kids, the tears are mostly because they are a big reason why fighting for my life was so critical. I will be here for them. I'm not going to let anything stand in my way.

Slowly it's formulating in my head what exactly this whole experience has boiled down to. Big changes. Simple changes.

I earned being done with chemo. I deserve feeling better now. I'll just never forget what I owe back to the rest of you. The truth is we aren't mean to go through life alone, we are meant to rely on each other. It's the only way and now I understand that.

Family

Feb 11, 2011 5:42pm

I really don't mind being sick here and there if it means I leave the bathroom only to find Steve and the kids up in their bedroom laughing and giggling, putting PJ's on and just generally being silly. Or if it means coming back to the Family room where America's Funniest Home videos are on TV and everyone is laughing so hard there are tears coming down their eyes. The occasional nauseous pang really sort of fades away quickly when you're too busy enjoying life. I even don't mind waking up at the crack of dawn to Lucy saying "Time to get up Mommy, it's six-dot-dot-eleven".

I'm posting some photos from these past couple of days. I've learned to really like 'right now'. Take care!

A new beginning—my last entry

Feb 12, 2011 11:56am

There comes a time for things to end and new beginnings to take place and I sense it's that time for me. From now on I'll see my life as "before" and "after" all this. And these past 8 months as the transition between these two major chapters. As much as it's been wonderful to go through these changes with all of you, as much as it's been a wonderful support system for me, it's also true that one must at some point return to Life especially as my health challenges subside. Return to a new life, with new powerful insights and live them simply. I'd hate to become one of those people who have a lot to say to other people but forget to actually honor the message. It's time for me to ride off into the sunset and struggle to maintain what I learned.

There's no real magic to all this living business yet we make it so complicated sometimes. There is one truth from which all other insights seem to emanate. For me, the discovery that I am exactly where I am supposed to be was powerful. I'm not supposed to have more money right now. I'm not supposed to have a better car. I'm not supposed to be a different type of parent. And I'm not supposed to never have had cancer. Every little thing that happens is supposed to happen and we then have the free will to accept it and learn from it . . . or not and remain stuck in endless frustration, desire for something else and totally missing the lessons that can in fact lead us to an even better life. Accepting today somehow causes silly frustrations to fade away. Accepting today opens up the opportunity for forgiveness, a necessary requirement for peace of mind and freedom from anger and fear. Accepting today allows us to truly find joy in what is right under our noses. And then the clarity to change and adapt . . .

You'll note that these past 8 months have not been about cancer at all. None of this is about cancer. Cancer was a casual bystander in what has happened for me. I literally learned nothing new about cancer from the day of my diagnosis until today. I can barely articulate all the parameters of my type of breast cancer. It's a triple negative with a pile of other things that I honestly don't know. They're just not important. I knew enough to understand my treatment options but even those were always laid out so clearly for me. I let go of control and allowed life and the best hospital in the world to show me my options. The best choice was always obvious to me so I took it. But no, this isn't about cancer. None of what I've written is for cancer patients exclusively. It's for any human being who realizes that the gems we are provided in life are already right in our hands. We all experience fear, pain, joy, loss and deciding how to live within that is the challenge we all face. Some of us ignore that fact and some of us search for the answer.

Thank you for listening to me as I found my version of the answer. I hope you also find yours.

See you in the real world. God Bless.

Epilogue

Life doesn't end when you are diagnosed with cancer and it also doesn't go back to "normal" when the treatments are all done. I will never be the same person I was before and hopefully I am kinder, gentler, more forgiving and more grown up.

I don't know what the future holds but I do know that I will no longer wait to do the things that matter and no longer waste my time and energy on the wrong things. I would rather only live 5 more years as I am living now than having gone on 30 years unaware of the real joy of life. And I mean that . . .